A Survivor's Guide to Open Heart Surgery

Rick and Rose Froyd

Charlotte Community Library
Charlotte, MI 48813

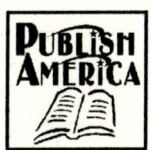

PublishAmerica
Baltimore

© 2002 by Almeda Rose Froyd and Donald R. Froyd, Jr.
All rights reserved. No part of this book may be reproduced in any form without written permission from the publishers, except by a reviewer who may quote brief passages in a review to be printed in a newspaper or magazine.

First printing

ISBN: 1-59286-019-2
PUBLISHED BY PUBLISHAMERICA BOOK PUBLISHERS
www.publishamerica.com
Baltimore

Printed in the United States of America

Acknowledgments

To Rose

Words simply cannot adequately express my profound sense of gratitude to you for your support, protection, compassion, and tireless diligence in taking care of me while I recovered from my surgery. Rose, I truly believe there is a beautiful crown awaiting you in heaven.

To Dennis Wong, Ph.D.

I consider you my mentor and friend. Your brilliance in clinical supervision is truly without peer. Your profound sense of ethical and compassionate approach to clinical work has deepened my respect for the wounded individual in both the clinical setting as well as every other aspect of life. I still marvel at the profound depth of the clinical supervision we went into! It is my continuing honor and privilege to know and communicate with you. I offer you my deepest thanks for your encouragement in this project.

To Renetta Williamson-Coe, MFT

You were so patient with me as I began my clinical work! Your careful and thoughtful approach to clinical work and clinical supervision still runs in my mind as I approach my own work. I so admire your tenacious adherence to solid theory and sound, ethical, clinical practice. You are so wonderful at teaching by example. You have my utmost respect.

Christine Heaney

Your enthusiasm and support for my writing projects are so energizing for me. Thank you so much for your editorial ideas and assistance. You are a true encourager and act as a positive catalyst for your supervisees, students and friends.

To Joe Hamilton, MFT

Your approach to clinical work has offered me an excellent exposure to a different theoretical view that is most interesting and is helping to round my clinical work. I am especially thankful for your encouragement with this project and the resources that you helped make me aware of. I am also thankful for your sage advice on achieving a better understanding of operating in governmental business systems.

Preface

Open-chest heart surgery is, in my opinion, one of the most dramatic surgeries a person can have. These surgeries are most often performed for Coronary Artery Bypass Grafting (CABG) or Valve replacement, such as in the case of Valvular disease. Exacerbating the drama is the fact that the patient must undergo heart-lung bypass and have their hearts stopped for a time while the surgeons perform the repairs. It is an awesome thing for the patient to consider having this surgery performed on his body, and incredibly difficult for his family members to grapple with as well.

This book is intended to be a helpful resource to heart patients who have already had their surgeries, hopefully validating some of their experiences, to heart patients who are facing this surgery in the future, and to the families of those patients who are trying to understand what the surgery means to them as well.

When I underwent my open-chest heart surgery on December 21, 2000, my wife and I had approximately 40 hours, or just about two days, in which to prepare for this life and death drama. We had no one to call who was knowledgeable about heart surgery; our medical staff as wonderful as they were, did not spend any time talking with us about the process except to say that they would use a St. Jude's mechanical heart valve and that I would be "good as new in six months." We were literally in shock prior to the surgery, and for a significant time after the surgery. It would have been so welcome to have someone who had previously been through this experience to talk with, or to read a book such as this in order to be more informed about the process during those surreal hours prior to the procedure!

This book details the process step by step, and hopefully will be a helpful resource for other families who will be undergoing the procedure in their futures. As a unique feature, in some chapters I will be covering certain elements of the process of having open-chest heart surgery using some of my own experiences in office visits with doctors, communication difficulties with medical helpers and other experiences in an effort to prepare the reader for a wide variety of situations in their journey. I wish you all peace, health, and success.

Rick Froyd, M.A., August 2001

Chapter 1

Specifically Identifying the Kind of "Heart Disease" You Have

The American Heart Association (AHA) explains that "cardiovascular diseases account for about 950,000 deaths annually (about 41 percent of total mortality from all causes). These diseases as a whole represent the No. 1 cause of death in the United States" (American Heart Association Heart and Stroke 2000 Statistical Update). More specifically, cardiovascular heart disease is responsible for "about 460,000 deaths annually."

Myocardial Infarction (MI) (Or "Heart Attack"):
In recognizing the symptoms of heart disease, the American Heart Association indicates that there are certain diagnostic features peculiar to heart disease, such as:

Classic Warning Signs:

- Uncomfortable pressure, fullness, squeezing or pain the center of the chest that lasts more than a few minutes, or goes away and comes back.
- Pain that spreads to the shoulders, neck or arms.
- Chest discomfort with lightheadedness.

Less Common Warning Signs:

- Atypical chest pain, stomach or abdominal pain.
- Nausea or dizziness (without chest pain).

- Shortness of breath and difficulty breathing (without chest pain.)
- Palpitations, cold sweat or paleness.

Special Note:
The AHA further relates, "not all of these warning signs occur in every heart attack. Sometimes they go away and return. If some occur, get help fast."

Those folks having an MI most generally are having problems with their coronary arteries, the arteries that supply the heart with the blood it needs to perform its rather formidable task of continuously pumping your life-blood throughout your body for your entire life. For reasons as much genetic as bad diets, the arteries become severely narrowed or blocked and do not allow enough blood to pass through them to supply the heart with vital nutrients to keep it nourished while pumping. This results in heart failure. The physicians and surgeons use a standardized and recognized classification system called the New York Heart Association Classification. According to the Heart Failure Society of America, "in order to determine the best course of therapy, physicians often assess the stage of heart failure according to the New York Heart Association (NYHA) functional classification system. This system relates symptoms to everyday activities and the patient's quality of life." In their wonderful web site, they explain the classes as follows:

- Class I is considered mild and there is no limitation of physical activity. Ordinary physical activity does not cause any problems
- Class II the person has a slight limitation of physical activity. Ordinary physical activity results in fatigue, palpitation, or dyspnea (shortness of breath)
- Class III the person has marked limitation of physical

activity. Comfortable at rest, but less than ordinary activity causes fatigue, palpitation, or dyspnea (shortness of breath)
- Class IV the person is unable to carry out any physical activity without discomfort. Symptoms of cardiac insufficiency at rest. If any physical activity is undertaken, discomfort is increased.

It seems that the American Heart Association has done a splendid job of informing the general public of the danger signals of an MI or heart attack. In my own experience, I had been very familiar with these symptoms; however, my heart problem did not have any of these signs until two days before my angiogram. In fact, the only symptom I had was shortness of breath and severe fatigue. I had a different form of heart disease: Aortic Valve Disease culminating in Class III Heart Failure.

Diagnosing a Heart Attack

There are a number of different diagnostic tools used to detect heart problems. Some of these tests are well known, such as the angiogram and the chest X-ray. However, there are some newer technologies that are making very accurate pictures of targeted areas inside the body and are being used by more and more cardiologists and cardiac surgeons. Please refer to the AHA publication, "Heart and Stroke Facts."

Treating Heart Attacks

The treating cardiologist will perform a thorough examination using the tests that he or she thinks is necessary. If it is determined that the heart attack was caused by blockages in the coronary arteries that supply blood to the heart itself, the doctor will determine if the blockages are of such a degree that they can be sufficiently cleared using tools in the angiography room. Some of these procedures are balloon angioplasty, laser angioplasty, atherectomy, a stint procedure, and finally coronary artery bypass grafting (CABG). In all of these procedures except the "bypass" procedure, the instrument is inserted most often into a large blood vessel in the patient's leg and guided into the heart. The cardiologist then manipulates the instrument into the damaged coronary artery and performs the procedure.

In balloon angioplasty, a "balloon" tip is used on the surgical instrument and inserted into the collapsing or clogged coronary artery and inflated. In doing this, the plaque is compressed and the vessel's diameter is enlarged.

In laser angioplasty, the tip of the instrument has a laser device on it and when inserted into the compromised coronary artery, emits light pulses that destroy the plaque.

An atherectomy involves having a shaving device or "burr" on the end of the catheter and grinding the plaque into extremely small particles.

The stint is a device that is implanted in the coronary artery to keep it open.

Coronary Artery Bypass Grafting (CABG) is an open-chest heart surgery performed by a cardiac surgeon. If this procedure is used, then the blockage of the coronary arteries was determined to be beyond the scope of angioplasty intervention.

During the procedure, the cardiac surgeon reroutes blood around the blocked arteries using veins from the patient's body, most often a vein from the leg or breast. Much of the personal story given below will apply to the CABG patient as well since they go through virtually the same process as the valve replacement patient except the area on the heart which is operated upon.

Valvular Disease

In explaining Aortic Valve disease, we must identify what a heart valve is and what it does. The heart has four chambers:

right and left atriums, and the right and left ventricles. Without getting too technical, each chamber has a valve between them, the mitral valve, the aortic valve, the tricuspid valve and the pulmonary valve. Valves have either a bicuspid or tricuspid presentation, or basically two flaps or three flaps. These valves close as the blood pumps through the heart to prevent the blood from backing up or going the wrong way in the system and open when the blood must pass through the heart.

A "stenotic" valve is malformed by lesions, calcium deposits or both and operates so that when it is open; it only opens a very small amount, which makes it difficult for an adequate amount of blood to go through to the next chamber. The cause is speculated to be either a birth defect or by an untreated disease such as rheumatic fever.

A valve with regurgitation is basically the opposite of stenosis: regurgitation means that the cuspids or leaflets of the valve do not close sufficiently enough for the hemodynamics of the heart to perform properly. In other words, the regurgitated blood has a "back-flow" and makes the ventricle in the heart work extra hard to pump blood through it. This causes the heart chamber associated with the regurgitation to become enlarged by its efforts to pump harder.

According to some data, most often, the Aortic Valve is replaced in men, and the Mitral Valve is replaced in women. However, it seems that women tend to have more Double Valve Replacements (DVR), where both the aortic and the mitral valves are replaced in the same procedure.

However, the American Heart Association indicates, "The NHLBI's Framingham Heart Study reports that prevalence is about 1-2 percent and no more common in women than men. This was a study of people ages 26-84" (American Heart Association Heart and Stroke 2000 Statistical Update). It seems that more research data need to become available before a more accurate picture of the gender issue can be confidently identified.

Warning Signs and Symptoms

According to the AHA, "the symptoms vary greatly from person to person. Often the damage to heart valves isn't immediately noticeable." Most often, the doctor will listen to your heart and notice a "click" or "murmur." This will be the beginning of a monitoring process. As the disease progresses, the patient may notice a gradual decrease in the ability to tolerate exercise. In my own case, I had adapted to the symptoms to such a degree that I was still working out six months before it became acutely difficult to get out of bed, although as I look back, it was getting very hard to get a good work out in.

Treatment

It is very important for patients with a heart murmur to take prophylactic antibiotics prior to any surgery or dental procedures. The reason for this is that any outside bacteria getting into the bloodstream can become lodged on the defective heart valve and cause more damage that will result in valve failure or a serious life-threatening infection.

When the heart valve becomes unable to perform its function properly, surgery is indicated. There are three basic replacement options: (1) a human donor valve, (2) a porcine (pig) valve, or (3) an artificial or mechanical valve. This is open-chest heart surgery.

Arrhythmias

The AHA states that arrhythmias are abnormal heart rhythms, which can cause the heart to pump less effectively. In a normal event, the heartbeat starts in the right atrium when cells send an electrical signal. These cells spread throughout the atria cells and follow down to the ventricles. The atria contract a split second before the ventricles. This begins your specific rhythm and should repeat exactly as before to have a "normal" rhythm.

Any change in the above-mentioned results is an arrhythmia. The AHA states that an arrhythmia can occur when:

1. The heart's natural pacemaker develops an abnormal rate or rhythm.
2. The normal conduction pathway is interrupted, or
3. Another part of the heart takes over as pacemaker

Some signs or symptoms of arrhythmias as noted by the AHA are:

- Bradycardias or slow pumping, fatigue, dizziness, lightheadedness, fainting or near fainting spells or even death.
- Tachycardias or rapid pumping, palpitations, rapid heart action, shortness of breath, chest pain, dizziness, lightheadedness, fainting or near fainting.
- Ventricular fibrillation, which is an extremely fast, chaotic rhythm during which the lower chambers quiver and the heart can't pump any blood. Cardiac arrest, collapse and sudden death follow unless medical help is provided immediately.

Treatment
Most arrhythmias are treated with medications or pacemakers.

Angina Pectoris
The AHA says that this is a term for chest pain due to coronary heart disease. The main reason for the pain in the chest event is that the heart is not getting enough blood to

supply its own oxygen needs. Angina is one of the classic warning signs of a heart attack.

Treatment
The administration of "vasodilators," or drugs that cause the blood vessels to relax and open are usually prescribed. Additionally, Nitroglycerin is used which relaxes the veins, which, in turn eases the heart's workload.

Congenital Heart Diseases
There are a number of conditions present at birth and are listed in the AHA booklet, "Heart and Stroke Facts." Simply call their toll-free telephone number and they will send the information you request right to your home.

Important Statistical Information
Other important statistics from the American Heart Association state that Congestive Heart Disease (CHD) is:

- The single largest killer of American males and females
- About every minute someone will die from a coronary event
- About 220,000 people a year die of CHD without being hospitalized. Most of these are sudden deaths caused by cardiac arrest, usually resulting from ventricular fibrillation (AHA, Heart and Stroke 2000 Statistical Update)

It should be noted here that there are many different complications that can require heart surgery, such as coronary artery disease, valvular disease, deformities of the septum, and congestive heart failure. The AHA numbers indicate that the two most prominent procedures are valve replacements (89,000 in 1999), and bypass (553,000 in 1999). The AHA is approximately two years behind in publishing statistics as a part of their statistical formulations so these are the most current data I could obtain.

Clearly, heart disease is an incredibly significant issue in this country and while it seems that technology is marching forward making stunning successes in the physical repairs of the body, I have yet to encounter any substantive literature on the emotional aftermath of such surgeries on the patient and their families.

Chapter 2

A Personal Account of the Diagnostic Process, Surgical Procedure, and Recovery

Now that we have identified the basic areas of the heart that receive surgical procedures, let us examine how these diseases are diagnosed. I remember how reading statistics on heart disease or cancer prior to my own experience was somewhat a "matter-of-fact experience." I remember thinking, "How difficult it must be for the person and their families when they are told." I never thought I would be the one to experience that tragic news.

I have always considered myself to be very healthy for the majority of my life. I exercised regularly with weights and performed some "cardio" on the bicycles in the gym. However, during the year prior to my surgery I began to slow down on working out. I had no idea that it was due to my heart failing. My wife and daughter would remark that I seemed to be "sleeping my life away." Somewhat of an exaggeration of my need for naps on a daily basis and sleeping in on the weekends. I just did not have the stamina that I normally had.

During my initial four years in the U.S. Air Force, a flight surgeon denied my request for "flight duty" because he found a "heart murmur." I was 22 years old at the time. The surgeon told me that it would "probably never bother me." After a brief interlude in the civilian sector, I rejoined another military organization and spent fifteen years there. During the physicals in this period, no mention of a heart murmur was made to me except on my last two visits before getting out.

Twelve months prior discharge, a physician's assistant noted a "heart murmur" but did not tell me. I later found out after examining my medical records that she had, in fact, recommended an echocardiogram at that time. The medical personnel who were responsible for handling my medical records and care failed to schedule the "echo." Additionally, a very thoughtful doctor in a subsequent medical examination noted a "click" as he listened to my heart and told me that my heart murmur "does not seem too serious," and that I would probably "outlive most of my peers." He said that it was Mitral Valve Prolapse, a condition that is "not serious at all." Sadly, he did not order an echocardiogram either.

As a normal course of getting out of the military, I went through a Veteran's Administration disability evaluation process and requested an echo for my heart murmur. This doctor was obviously not interested in listening to my heart. He listened for a quick minute and then replied, "Your heart murmur is not serious enough to warrant an echo, but you should get one for your own peace of mind by your private physician." I did just that. I went to my primary care provider who happens to be one of the most thorough and knowledgeable doctors I have ever met. This doctor referred me to a cardiologist who had a technician perform the echocardiogram. It took almost 14 days to get the results so I thought the test was "normal." After all, they call when things are not normal, don't they? Evidently the cardiologist's office was extra busy or unable to turn tests around quickly—even tests with serious disease processes identified. I will never forget that moment. The doctor looked at the results and I could see the expression on his face change. He looked at me and said, "Rick, you wanted an evaluation of your mitral valve prolapse, but I am afraid that you have a much more serious condition than that."

Of course, I began to feel somewhat dissociated from the event as each moment passed. The doctor continued, "Look at this report with me, your aortic valve has a lot of calcium on it and it is not closing properly." The report went on to state that I must be monitored by echocardiogram every three months and begin vasodilator therapy to help with blood flow. There was notice of the enlargement of my left ventricle, the "main pumping chamber of the heart," and a moderate to severe regurgitation, or blood flow going the opposite way in the system. This was a scant three months after the VA doctor listened to my heart.

It is not my intention to consign unanswered or undue blame upon this VA doctor or the Veterans Administration. However, after consultation with my heart surgeon, my primary care physician, and my cardiologist, it was agreed by all that my condition had to have been eminently noticeable during my last years in the military organization. I am deliberately not naming the "military" organization mostly because of my negative experiences with them and consequent negative view I have of them as a "military" organization. In other words, my view is somewhat biased and probably not fair to that organization.

I decided to write about my own personal experience with the diagnostic aspect of heart disease, primarily because, if mistakes happened in my care, it has happened or is happening to someone else, either in the military or civilian sectors. In the current medical and mental health climate of managed care, understaffed medical offices and cost conscious care giving, patients have the very important task of being their own advocate. Potential heart patients ignore this reality at their own peril.

I would speculate that if I had not initiated the request for an echocardiogram, my family and I might have taken a trip in our motor home to a secluded place as we often do, and I may have died leaving a stunned and helpless wife in a very difficult position. Prior to my surgery, I slept soundly. I had no idea that I was just days, possibly hours close to death.

The most concerning thing for my wife was that she could not "get me out of bed," I just wanted to sleep. Only two days prior to my surgery did I become noticeably short of breath, and this was only for a short time. This was not so clearly a sign of heart disease for me; you see, I have asthma. A different scenario would have been that I would have had to make an unscheduled trip to the emergency room via ambulance, and they would have performed open-chest heart surgery on me without any preparation at all. This is undesirable for at least two reasons: my wife would be exposed to more intense shock without any support from family during the surgery, and it would be very surprising to wake from surgery with a cracked chest, hooked up to all of the monitoring equipment, especially the tubes coming from the chest, and being so helpless.

The above scenarios can all be avoided if the patient is informed about heart disease and how to be their own advocate. However, there are some circumstances where the surgery must be performed on an emergency basis and cannot be put off for the patient to "get prepared."

Once I called my cardiologist and explained that I was having shortness of breath and fatigue, he asked if I would like to have an angiogram. I replied yes. He mentioned to me that he was not "impressed with my symptoms" as I was describing them to him.

I remember feeling shame at having to say, "Something is wrong with me and I need help." Chances are some of you reading this book may feel this same way, please stand up for yourself and be counted—it is probably better for you and your family if you "complain a little too much" than dismiss something gravely wrong. Again, if you have a deep concern that something is wrong with you, strenuously voice this to your doctors. At some point, the communication will connect and the problem will be either identified or absolutely disproved.

I would like to mention one more instance of where physicians and work colleagues were not listening to someone in trouble. I held a supervisor position for some time during my military career. I had been assigned a young woman who was being described as "constantly getting into trouble and has an attitude." As I began to listen to this person, she was indeed under a lot of stress, but I was convinced there was something physically wrong going on with her. After months of me encouraging her to "keep after those doctors" and her being harassed and given poor evaluations by an uninformed and inexperienced junior officer, this woman was literally just about to give up. But she kept telling the doctors that "something was wrong" with her. Ultimately, they found a tumor in her brain. It was benign, but located in a place that could compromise some of her autonomic functioning. I took her to the hospital the day of check-in, as no family was there for her at that time. At my last contact with her, the surgery was successful.

Back to my own situation, the echocardiogram was an easy procedure. All I had to do was lie on a table and the technician hooked me up with wires, placed the conducting gel on my chest, and began to take pictures. There was no discomfort at all. However, the angiogram was a different story.

As a diagnostic tool, the angiogram seems to be the preferred and most accurate tool in the cardiologist's tool bag. The cardiologist can get hyper-accurate information about blood flow ejection fractions, coronary artery blockage percentages, and measurements of enlarged chambers. They can also perform certain surgical procedures that include balloon angioplasty and the implantation of stints (referred to in an earlier chapter).

The Angiogram Procedure

I was admitted to a day surgery clinic at a hospital in my

hometown. Incidentally, this hospital's heart program was recently recognized as one of the top hospitals in a recent study performed by the HCIA-Sachs "100 TOP Hospitals: Cardiovascular Benchmarks for Success study in 1999." This procedure was performed in a special operating room that has specific equipment for an angiogram. I was given a sedative and prepared for the insertion of a catheter that can contain instruments that would enter into a large artery in my right groin area and be carefully guided to my heart to perform their tasks. I must say that the thought of this procedure gave me much anxiety. I expected to have more pain, but luckily, my cardiologist was good at numbing the site of insertion.

During this procedure, he measured my blood flow through my aortic valve and also examined other features of my heart condition such as: coronary artery functioning, left ventricle enlargement, and ejection fraction. The worst part of the procedure for me was when he released the dye into my veins. The doctor said, "Now you will feel something warm." Well, it was not "warm," it was just plain hot, and it made me feel anxious. The cardiologist also explained, "Now you will feel your heart skip a beat."

I did feel this as well. It is a strange and anxiety-provoking thing to have someone manipulating your heart while you are awake. However, I am grateful for the technology and the people who endeavor to gain such expertise and use it for healing purposes.

As I was having this procedure performed, my wife Rose entered the room where the cardiologist was examining the data. Rose related that this doctor showed her the results of the blood flow measurements and said to her, "Your husband is not going to die *today*, but he needs surgery by the end of the week—I am paging the cardiac surgeon now." He also said, "You and Mr. Froyd have a lot to discuss." Rose asked if he had told me yet and he replied, "No." She remembers being disappointed that the doctor chose not to talk to me himself and he put it all on her. Meanwhile, I was still lying flat on the procedure table, a medical technician applying direct pressure on the large insertion point in my groin artery.

I was moved to the cardiac floor to lie flat for approximately four hours until the artery was able to clot.

I went for my angiogram on Tuesday, December 19, 2000. I was subsequently scheduled for open-chest heart surgery on December 21, 2000 at 7:30 a.m. The next day and a half would be filled with many thoughts and emotions.

Although I am a therapist and have a desire and habit to use introspection and reflection, I found myself being torn toward dissociation, or a state of "psychic numbing" or "zoning out." I remember thinking, "I'm only 40 years old, I have worked out all of my adult life, and now I have to have heart surgery—this can't be."

I can imagine two different scenarios where someone in this situation would struggle with this dilemma:

Healthy Life Style	**Less Healthy Life Style**
The person who has worked out regularly three or more times a week, was careful about what kinds of food they ate, and limited the amount of the "bad" fats in their diet. **Feelings** This person is bound to feel on a continuum, maybe beginning with exasperation, then to anger, and then to rage. They might think to themselves, "…I have done all of the right things…" This person may also feel like giving up since what the "experts said" did not work for them.	This category applies to the person who rarely or never worked out, and may have smoked cigarettes. This person probably drank a little too much and ate whatever they felt like eating without attention to fat, sugars, or any other diet information. **Feelings** This person may feel shame about their condition and may feel as if they brought it on themselves. They may have a family member(s) that is/are so angry with them that they are getting in their "I told you so's."

> **Feelings are a normal part of this process**
>
> However, I do not recommend beating yourself up because of your heart condition, nor do I recommend that you allow someone else to beat you up over it. Instead, it is my experience that you allow yourself to "get in touch" with your situation "in the moment." In other words, you or someone you love or care about has heart disease, use human love, concern, and comfort during this time, not finger pointing or self-recrimination to deal with your disease process. Because ultimately, we live or die with our actions. How do you want to be remembered? Or people to remember you?

I wanted to run from this whole thing; pretend that it was not happening. I remember feeling a great need to have "closure" with the people in my life in some way. There wasn't time to speak with everyone. However, I was able to call many of the people whom I cared about. I called and told them of my imminent surgery and that if anything should happen and I died, that I wanted them to know how much they meant to me and how they had impacted my life.

Not all of my communications were pleasant ones. I grew up in a severely alcoholic home. I remember grieving especially hard on December 20, 2000 for the father that I never had. I wished so much that I could have spent a few hours talking with a father who had been there for me as I grew up, encouraging me, teaching me, role modeling appropriate behaviors for me. Sadly, I never had that. It would have been such a comfort for me during the time prior to surgery to share my fears with a father. I sent my family a letter and shared with them how disappointed I was in the alcoholism and dysfunction in the family as I grew up. This caused quite a stir as you might imagine. No matter how much of a stir that I caused, I still think I did the right thing.

My goal was to share my honest feelings and thoughts, as I never could before due to the communication dysfunction inherent in my "family of origin." However, some would say that what I did was a bit harsh. Nonetheless, this is one of those decisions one must make for oneself.

My wife was wonderful during this time. She allowed me the space I needed to reflect on my life and relationships, and we also came together and comforted each other. We have both lived as a military family moving up and down the west coast for 15 of our 17 years of marriage, and so we were used to times of being alone as a couple. But looking back, I wish that we would have reached out more to our friends and my wife's family for support. As it was, Rose had to wait in the hospital alone during my surgery; a dreadful task I would not wish on any person.

I checked into the hospital on Wednesday, December 20, 2000 at 12:00 p.m., and was assigned to the cardiac unit. Instead of getting more anxious or at least becoming more aware of my anxiety, I found the situation becoming more surreal. It would have been wonderful to have someone explaining the process that would take place over the next few hours and days, but none was forthcoming. Eventually two nurses showed up and began to shave all of the hair from my chest and legs. They used battery-operated clippers that pulled the hair. This was very uncomfortable. If I had to do it all over again, I would have shaved myself prior to going to the hospital. But then, I wasn't told that I would need to be shaved. I would also add that I could have stopped the nurses and required them to find a less painful way; however, I was not aware yet that I was responsible for being my own advocate.

The patient can say, "No."

Next they gave me a "special" soap that I would shower with the night before surgery, and again in the morning just before being taken to the operating room. I remember feeling so out of place. Prior to being shaved, my body was moderately hairy; it no longer looked like my own body. The shower ritual reminded me of passages that I had read about the Nazi concentration camps. I was thinking some very morbid thoughts.

Dinner was served but neither Rose nor I were very hungry. Later that evening the anesthesiologist came to my room to discuss the particulars of my case. He was very nice and we were able to laugh with him a little. In fact, Rose and I still giggle about our visit with him. He assured me that I would not "wake up" during the surgery, and that I would not feel a thing.

On the evening of the 20th, Rose and I kissed good night, she left for home and I was given something to "help me sleep." I was awakened early the next morning, asked to shower once again with the special soap and allowed to drink water. I was given another sedative to help with relaxation. Rose arrived to see me off to the operating room. The ride down to the operating room was another surreal experience. The first person that I met in the operating room was the familiar (covered) face of the anesthesiologist. He had a needle in his hand as he was reaching for my hand. I remember saying to him, "Hey, the medicine you gave me is not really relaxing me." This is that last thing I can remember until waking up in the cardiac ICU.

Open-Chest Heart Surgery

I cannot write about my own open-chest heart surgery since I was obviously under very powerful anesthesia. But during this time, Rose recalls waiting in a designated waiting room for surgery patients. She was assigned to a nurse whose duty it was to follow two heart surgery patients. The nurse would come out and tell Rose when I was placed on the bypass machine, and then again when I came off the bypass machine. Rose told me afterwards that this was quite possibly the hardest waiting time she had ever gone through. She felt few people could really be of help during this time for her.

I had gone into surgery at 7:00 a.m., and I awoke in the Cardiac ICU some time around 1:30 p.m., on the same day. I was in quite a fog, but I remember asking the ICU nurse what was wrong. I was trying to ask her, "Why are you so nervous?" Since I had tubes running out of practically every orifice of my body and I was on a ventilator, Rose suggested that she let me write what I needed to say. I guess my first attempt at writing was pretty bad—they asked me to "slow down and try it again." I wrote, "What is wrong?" Rose stayed with me during most of my ICU stay, and she said that this particular nurse was the most vigilant and compassionate nurse that she had ever seen. The nurse said to me that I had to try and remember to breathe because if I didn't, the machine would alarm. I remember being satisfied at their answer, and then I drifted in and out until the next day at around 1:00 p.m.

At this time, a different ICU nurse began to disconnect me from all of the tubes and the ventilator. I remember feeling very vulnerable and frightened. I remarked to Rose, "I don't trust this guy."

It could be that I am stereotyping men and women, or it could be that men represent more of a threat at a basic level to my unconscious than do women, or it could just be that this particular nurse emitted a negative energy. I am a trained therapist, and I did not see any compassion in the eyes of this caregiver—it was very disconcerting. Whatever it was, it was very uncomfortable to be at the whim of someone I did not trust when my chest had been literally sawed open, wired and glued together and one soft movement could cause immense pain and significant bodily damage. I do not think I have ever felt as defenseless as I did at that time.

Thankfully, Rose was there to observe the process of this nurse removing my tubes and equipment. She was a real advocate for me; she said that she had to practically grab this person by the throat to get me a warm blanket while he was leaving me exposed for periods of time. If you are going to have heart surgery, try your best to have someone who is strong willed accompany you throughout the surgery; you definitely need an advocate when you cannot be one for yourself.

The Recovery Process Begins
Once I had been unhooked and it was ascertained that I could breathe on my own, I was placed in a less intense level of care on the Cardiac Care Unit. It was here, when they shifted me from the mobile gurney to my bed, that I discovered how incredibly painful it was to move. The other medication was probably wearing off as well. I have no misgivings about letting doctors, dentists, or other health care professionals know if I am in pain. They knew in a hurry that I was uncomfortable. I asked for Demerol. However, they administered morphine.

For some reason, morphine does not work as efficiently for me; something my vital signs showed as my skyrocketing heart rate and blood pressure attested to. I did get Demerol for the first day, but after that, I was to take Vicodin.

I have worked in a Hospice setting where pain management is viewed very differently than in the traditional medical community. I remember being exceedingly upset that I was not getting the kind of pain management I wanted. I was in constant, chronic pain, which was lessened by the Vicodin, but by the third hour after administration, I was fit to be tied. The nursing staff would tell me, "It is not time for your meds yet." I would literally demand Demerol, a medication that really seemed to help with the pain, but they would explain that I would not heal properly if I took that medication. I would later do some of my own research on the use of pain medication during recovery from open-chest heart surgery. My research reveals that I should have been given the Demerol for at least the first few days.

The CCU staff would ask me to cough, to get up and walk around, and to keep an oxygen candela under my nose. The oxygen dried my nose out to the point of bleeding. Coughing was particularly painful as you can imagine, but they gave me a heart-shaped pillow to hold tightly against my chest while I coughed. The coughs were deep and full of fluid. This fluid was from the bypass machine. After the surgery, it was explained to me that in order to begin the process of the machine taking over the circulation for my body, they "primed" it with a type of saline solution. Some of this solution gets into the lungs and one must "cough it out" after the surgery. Sadly, I also suffer from asthma and the solution somehow exacerbated this asthmatic condition resulting in a very serious day or two of extremely labored breathing.

Friends and family who visited during this time thought that I was probably going to die. So did I. I desperately wanted to die to stop the pain; to avoid being out of work, to avoid how my life would probably change drastically from the life I once knew.

It was on this day, day three after surgery that I announced rather matter-of-factly, "I am not going to cough today, nor am I going to walk today, and I want everyone to leave me alone." Rose asked me if I wanted her to go home and I replied, "Yes." I then turned the thermostat in my room up to almost maximum and lay down to sleep. I was so miserable! All I wanted to do was die. I cannot remember if Rose contacted staff on her way out, or if she did it after leaving for an hour or two and coming back to the hospital. But she told my nurse that she thought I was going to give myself a fever and that I was trying to die. Well, in comes this wonderful certified nurse's assistant. She barked out orders better than any boot camp drill instructor that I ever heard: "This room is too hot, you need to get up and walk, and I'm not taking no for an answer."

I told her no. But she turned the thermostat down herself, took my covers down and began to pull me up. I grumbled and groaned and we went for a walk. We argued about my lack of pain medication and other material that I simply cannot remember at this point, for the entire walk. If I could see this saint again, I would give her the biggest hug and "thank you" that I could. Somehow, she played a critical role in my recovery process and I am not sure just what it was. Maybe it was just that she cared enough to struggle with me. Maybe it was that she provided a solid shoulder at a moment when I needed it. Maybe it was because she was not intimately involved with me and so she could just be neutral about "kicking me in the butt."

A lung specialist was called in to treat my asthma condition. I recall this man looking over at me as I lay breathing out popping, wheezing, and gasping sounds. I remember he looked so kind and concerned as he leaned over my bed and talked to me. He had been a doctor for many years, and I later found out that he would be retiring a year after my surgery. I find it amazing that he still cared so much for humans in pain, even though he was in a life stage where many people are "burned out" from their jobs. He explained, "I'm going to try some treatments for a few days, if your lung doesn't get any better, I might have to scope it." I said to him, "Doctor, I am tired of the pain; I would rather die than be subjected to chronically painful treatments." This was not an attempt at theatrics. I had had enough of the pain and deep breathing would only make my broken chest hurt more. I remember this with crystal clarity. He responded, "I'll use a ventilator that will gently put medicine into your lungs – if it hurts too much I will stop it." This was a critical moment in my healing process. Something that I wish I could lovingly intimate to the medical community—respect for human beings to make a choice.

Up to that point, the cardiac staff was ordering me around: "Cough, walk around, no Demerol, it's not time for your pain medicine yet, eat, and urinate!" This wonderful doctor actually had the respect for me to engage me in the treatment process by empowering me to say no when I needed to. I remember being aware at some level of consciousness, of being free to die if I needed to. I feel inadequate in being able to articulate the profundity of this shift in the treatment dynamic. I needed to be able to say, "no" when I wanted to.

I needed to be able to say, "It hurts" and receive medication for the pain. I needed to be able to remember that ultimately, it was between me and my God, whether I would be dying from this surgical procedure—not human intervention. Up to this point, human intervention, no matter how exquisitely professional and competent it was, only served to make me feel helpless and used. I recall asking God to "take me home" many times during my hospital stay and after I went home as well.

Alas, the breathing treatments were exceptionally painful for the next few days. I had lost almost all of the holding capacity for my lungs. The doctors gave me an air machine that measures lung capacity by blowing into it. I blew the little ball inside up to the top of the instrument and kept it there for many seconds effortlessly prior to the surgery. After the surgery, I could barely raise the ball inside to the first measurement.

I came to dread the respiratory therapists as they came by four times a day. They would connect me to a type of ventilator that blew medicine into my lungs. I remember being very careful on the first few measurements of how strong to set the machine—after all, my chest was extremely sensitive to movement. I hated the words, "okay, now cough." I wanted to run, I wanted out of that hospital as soon as possible. I am reminded how some respiratory therapist's (RTs) would literally "insist" that I work harder in the treatments. Whereas some would look at me in all of my pathetic glory and say, "Okay, you did good" as I protested after only a few breaths and they would leave me alone. I suppose I needed both types, but I just hated the breathing treatments.

Even after the forced breathing treatments were over, I had to continue with other contraptions to assist in my recovery from the asthmatic reaction well into the third month after treatment. As I write this, the dark feelings of just how difficult it was to struggle with breathing is as palpable today as it was back then.

For a time my oxygenation was below 80 percent. After the third day of treatment for the asthmatic condition, my body responded positively and began oxygenating to the level of 98 percent. This meant that I could take my candela off!

On approximately the sixth day of treatment, I was well enough for the physician's assistant to remove the chest tubes and electrical wires from my chest. It was explained to me that the tubes were placed in my chest cavity in the fat behind the ribs for the purpose of collecting the blood that might be oozing into it from the heart surgery. The pericardium, or the sack around the heart, is not sown all the way together after the surgery because fluids need to drain out of that area. If the fluids cannot escape, an infection will result which is very serious and could kill the patient. In my particular case of aortic valve replacement, after the heart is stopped, the chest clamp is in place and the patient is on the bypass machine, the aorta is then cut into above the heart in order for the surgeon to perform work on the valve just below the aorta inside the heart. The surgeon sutures the valve in place, and then he sutures the aorta back together, and drainage will also take place from these procedures.

Therefore, the surgeons placed two chest tubes that looked long and thin into my chest. The insertion points were just below the bottom of the chest incision. These tubes emptied their contents from the chest cavity into a box, much like the lunch box young children use to carry their lunches to school. Only these boxes had a side that was made of material that allowed its contents to be viewed from the outside. I remember watching all of the other heart patients and myself walking around the aisles carrying our blood boxes. It was a rather pitiful sight.

The physician's assistant who was following my case came in and remarked, "It's time to take your tubes and wires out." He appeared to me to be a short, wiry, "farm-raised boy." He explained that the wires in my chest were placed into my heart muscle and poked right through my chest skin for the purpose of optimum electrical stimulation in the event it was needed. He grabbed the wire and pulled quickly. He did this for both of the exposed wires. I felt queasy at the movement from deep inside my chest.

Next, he told me to brace myself as he was going to remove the drainage tubes placed in my chest. I asked for some painkillers, but he said it would be over before I knew it—so we should just get it over with. I should mention that I remember the tubes to be bigger around than a large sausage, and long enough to reach into my chest cavity. The surgeons during the surgery had made two small crosscuts in my belly just below my ribs where the tubes were, and the skin had begun to stick to the tubes. I took a deep breath and the physician's assistant put his leg up on the bed and quickly pulled the tubes out. I have never felt such an awful pain in my life. It felt as if he was pulling out all of the stuff inside me from my toes to my brain. The physician's assistant looked at me seemingly incredulously, like I was really acting out. I looked at him and said, "Don't other people think it's painful?" He replied, "Not that painful."

After the pulling out of my drainage tubes and several respiratory treatments, my chest was so painful that I asked the nurse if I had compromised my incision. She went and got that same physician's assistant! I was very reticent about relating to him what my concern was; however, I needed to have my incision checked out. Once again, he put a foot up on the bed and took his thumbs and began to push incredibly hard on each side of my incision from top to bottom. I screamed bloody murder! I remember saying, "Stop, I give up, I give up!" This particular incident grabbed the attention of the two rooms on either side of my room. I heard one of the patients ask the PA, "What the hell happened to *him*—you're not going to do that to *me* are you?"

The PA and I began to disagree on perceptions, and by the end of my stay in the hospital, he was openly wondering in front of the surgeon why the actual cardiac surgeon could lay his professional hand on my incision and ask me to cough and I could perform the task with bearable pain, and the PA could not. I replied, "The doctor does not hurt when he touches."

I sincerely hope that I was a factor in helping this young man learn how to have compassion for human beings. He seemed to still be in the stage of looking at patients as an amalgam of "systems" without notice of their humanity. That is my assumption. However, I believe that our actions and deeds speak much louder than our words and this man's actions spoke of harshness and blindness to individual humanness.

I used to think that it would be nice to stay in a hospital and be "taken care of." Well, it is difficult to get rested in a hospital. My day would start with being awakened at around 4:00 a.m. for a blood draw.

I recall one morning catching a young phlebotomist out of the corner of my half-asleep eyes hesitating on where to draw the blood from because there were so many needle marks, and then hesitating putting tape back on because my arms were looking pretty bad. I just was not up to suggesting that she not put any tape on. They needed to draw my blood every day to monitor my clotting factor to ensure that no blood clots formed on my new mechanical valve. They had to tape my arms after the blood draw and I also had tape on my stomach to hold tubing in place. I had a bad rash on both arms and stomach for weeks afterwards.

At 5:00 a.m. the X-ray technicians would come for me. They would help me out of the bed, which was dreadfully painful, and then into the wheelchair. The first two days after surgery I noticed that the wind would fly by my ears on these trips to the elevator and to the X-ray room. With a broken chest, this was concerning for me. However, after the first couple of days, I began to enjoy our race to the elevator. The technicians explained that they had to get a certain number of people done before a certain time. The X-ray folks were all young, very nice, even when they asked me to raise my hands above my head and all I could muster was about level with my shoulders with elbows in front!

> **Heparin** an anticoagulant. This is a more immediate acting drug that is injected subcutaneously in the stomach fat tissue every 12 hours during the first few days post surgery until stable INR is achieved.

After flying back from X-ray, I received a low sodium breakfast. The particular hospital that I was in had wonderful food! I really enjoyed the taste even if I could not eat it all in the first few days after surgery. After breakfast, the nurse would come in with a huge handful of pills to swallow. There were about eight pills in all, maybe more. Some pills were for my heart, some for skin, some for asthma, and some to help with pain. I wanted to know what each pill was and what it was supposed to do. I would also receive my subcutaneous heparin injection in my stomach, another blood-thinning agent to prevent clots on my valve.

I would then brush my teeth, wash my hands, and run water over my face. All of the television shows portray hospitalized people looking freshly showered and made up. It is not that way! If it were not for my wife, my hair would have been matted to my head. She would take waterless shampoo and wash my hair for me every evening. There was no way that I could shampoo my hair during the first few days after surgery, and quite frankly, the nurses did not volunteer to do this for me.

My next task was to walk around the corridor in order to strengthen the heart and improve vascular circulation. I began to enjoy this task, and would try to go one more lap than I did the day before. However, I shall never forget how all of a sudden I would become absolutely out of energy during the walks. Prior to surgery during workouts, I would be able to feel my body "winding down" slowly on energy after an hour or so. However, after surgery my body would lose its energy quite quickly leaving me helpless where I stood if I was not being helped by a nurse or my wife.

I would then need to rest and take a nap. After the nap, lunch would arrive and I would be given more pills. Throughout this time, I remember the Vicodin did not last the entire four hours and this was a constant source of irritation for me. I was not an ideal patient! After lunch, I would walk more, sneak decaf coffee from the nurses' station, and wonder why I was still alive.

I had a lot of time to contemplate this question and have yet to arrive at a satisfactory answer. I was becoming more depressed as the days went by and my own awareness was not catching it, nor was the medical staff. After all, I *was* taking an anti-depressant. Also throughout the day, I was still receiving breathing treatments.

Then dinnertime would arrive and I would eat. Rose would usually be at the hospital at this time. We would spend some hours together in the evening. I was not able to appreciate how difficult it must have been for her at that time due to my injuries. However, I am now, and she was and still is, a real angel.

During the dinner hour, I would be given the pills and the blood thinner shot in my stomach. Additionally, just after dinner I was receiving powerful intravenous antibiotics to prevent infection.

The surgeon's rounds seemed somewhat random. There would be morning rounds on some days, and evening rounds on others. I suppose that he would make rounds to fit his busy heart surgery schedule. This cardiac surgeon was extremely skilled and was very approachable and down to earth to my wife and me. The only thing that I knew about him was that prior to being recruited by the cardiac group, he had been on staff at the Mayo Clinic. I recall asking him at my pre-surgery visit, "How many valve replacements have you done?" He just looked calmly at me and after a brief pause replied, "Oh, hundreds." He placed a hand on my hand as if to reassure me that he was a definite professional.

During the rounds, he would sometimes ask me questions, or he would be getting information from two of the PA's. When my asthmatic lung began making trouble, he asked me, "Were you ever told that you had asthma?" I replied, "Yes." He then looked very thoughtful and announced to his staff with his finger in the air, "We will treat him as an asthmatic patient." I knew that I was in serious trouble, but I still got the biggest kick out of his remark. He seemed like one of those very brilliant people that are sometimes peculiarly animated. In any event, Rose told me that when the surgery was over and I was being taken to the ICU, this surgeon was kind enough to notice her in the hallway and make a point to speak with her. This may seem small, but to Rose it was very humane, respectful and needed at the time.

During day eight or the last day in the Cardiac Care Unit, the rounds were made and the PA explained that I was stable with the exception of my blood clotting (Prothrombin time [protime]/International Normalized Ratio [INR] factor). Therefore, it was recommended that I be moved to the skilled nursing facility in the same hospital until my PT/INR became stabilized.

If blood were to clot on the mechanical valve, it might prevent the valve from closing properly or opening properly. This would result in essentially the same condition that the valve was supposed to fix. Alternatively, the formed clot on the valve might become loose and move into another part of the body, such as the lung or brain and cause serious organ damage. Therefore, research has determined that the proper INR for a person with a mechanical heart valve should be between 2.5 and 3.5. There are other factors as well. For instance, if a person has clotted before, they prefer the INR to be a little higher. The patient is given the medication known as Coumadin (warfaran) for the purpose of causing the blood to clot less quickly. It takes some time for the medication to achieve "therapeutic levels" and so the injections of heparin, which act immediately and diminish after twelve hours, are used until the oral medication has obtained a stable level. Mine took a little time to achieve this stability. Even six months after surgery, I am still struggling to achieve a stable level.

> **Coumadin** or **Warfaran:** Essentially this drug prevents the blood from clotting quickly. Known as an anticoagulant. It usually takes two days to achieve stable levels in the body. It is commonly used as rat poison!

The skilled nursing facility was an even less intensive level of care than the Cardiac Care Unit. It appeared that this unit housed the chronically ill patients that were seriously ill and dying, or like me, needing to become stabilized in their current condition before leaving the hospital.

It was in this facility that I attempted my first shower. I recall that just getting my towels and toiletries together almost wore me out. Then it was down the hall to the showers. The shower stalls were lined with pink tiles from top to bottom.

As you might imagine, any little noise would echo rather easily in these stalls. This was the first time that my mechanical heart valve made its considerable impact on my soul. My pulse during those days measured between 80 and 90 beats per minute due to pain and activity intolerance. As I stepped into the shower, all I could hear was this quick-paced clicking. I remember experiencing an overabundance of feelings as my new heart valve reverberated away in the shower. I felt glad that my heart was "fixed." However, I also felt somewhat queasy that someone had invaded my physical body and placed a mechanical device inside me. It was foreign—I was no longer the person I once was, I was a heart surgery survivor. I felt a sense of grief over losing the idea of the healthy man I used to be. In addition, as curious as it seems, I felt a sense of grief or loss over losing my original heart valve. A very important piece of my body was now gone and replaced by a mechanical device.

As all of these feelings were encompassing my mind, I was attempting to perform a ritual that is almost subconscious—showering. I could only manipulate one hand at a time, and I could only raise one hand above my head. To use two hands would be too great a pressure on my chest incision. Just moving one hand was painful enough. Moreover, I was intensely afraid of falling down, so one hand held on to the shower faucet handles. Needless to say, I did not get as clean as I usually do after a shower that time, but at least I did rinse off with some soap. After all of this movement, I was so drained that I had to sleep for a couple of hours afterwards.

Release from the Hospital

Each day the PA's would be making rounds. My surgeon no longer accompanied the PA's on the rounds while I was in the skilled nursing facility. However, the PA would come by and ask me how I was doing and generally let me know that by their tests I was doing well, except they were trying to get my INR to the proper level. Finally, on the ninth day in the hospital, they came by and said that I could leave that afternoon. I recall getting the news just as they were beginning to hook me up to an intravenous antibiotic solution. They asked, "Do you want to go ahead and take the IV before you go?" I replied, "No thanks." I just wanted to get the heck out of there!

After signing a stack of paper inches thick, assuring the social worker that I could contact state disability by myself, and being notified that the in-home nursing staff would visit me for at least four weeks, I was wheeled downstairs to the main lobby. As the distinctive foyer came into my view, I remember thinking that I had not been sure that I would ever come this way again. Only here I was being wheeled to my waiting wife and car. Suddenly I became extremely concerned about being out in the world with a chest that had just been wired back together! The feeling was one of underlying panic.

Rose helped me into our beautiful blue Grand Marquis. I just loved this car and was glad that it had such a forgiving suspension system since every little bump in the road made a considerable impact on my incision. We only live a few miles from the hospital and Rose drove especially careful back to our place. We arrived at our new house and I began the process of "recovering" from heart surgery.

House-bound

Rose dropped me off at our house and took the prescriptions to the pharmacy to have them filled. There were so many of them! Not only were these medications foreign to us, they were having us use generic versus brand name, and then one was not available so the doctor's office had to be contacted to get further instruction. Both Rose and I were nervous about getting medicine that was not what the doctor ordered. Eventually Rose straightened it out with the doctors and the pharmacists. We have an island in our kitchen for the preparation of meals and such. We spread my medication out on this island and Rose wrote the times each were to be taken and their names. This became routine after the first few days.

We have a sofa in our living room that reclines on the ends and the middle pulls down where we can place our drinks and snacks. During the next four months of recovery, I would sleep on this recliner, as it was too uncomfortable for me to sleep on the bed. Rose slept on the recliner next to me because she said, "I found myself coming into the living room two or three times a night to see if you were still alive." I have never felt such a sense of warmth as when she did this. Every night there we were in our house, Rose watching over me vigilantly, and me helpless as a child.

Rose remembers that she would wake me up in the morning to take my medication and I would try to stay awake to visit with her. After she left, I would brush my teeth and take a shower. I was very aware that I had to be especially careful when showering; one slip and I could fall. Once my shower was over, I would be drained and need to rest for an hour or so.

For the first few weeks, I was recovering at home, part of my treatment plan included visits from a Home Health Nurse. My home health nurse was a wonderful, compassionate, knowledgeable Dutch woman who was extremely good at what she did. She would weigh me, check my ankles for swelling, draw blood for clotting measurements, take my blood pressure, and ascertain my own subjective opinion of my condition. The first few visits my pulse was between 80 and 100 beats per minutes and my blood pressure was sporadic. Prior to this surgery, my sitting pulse was around 65 to 70 beats per minute. However, eventually my vital signs evened out. She carefully questioned me about any adverse reactions to medications or if I were experiencing any problematic physical reactions related to the surgery. The only problem we figured out was that the Digitalis I was taking, designed to make the heart pump effectively, gave me periodic double vision. I remember looking forward to her visiting me and experiencing sadness on our last visit.

The first few weeks were mostly spent on eating, sleeping, showering, and visiting with Rose and with some friends on the telephone. After about eight weeks, I began to try sleeping on the bed, but it still hurt too much so I stayed on the recliner. I began to try walking short distances. I would get up every hour or so and walk around the front room, dining room, down the hall, and back into the front room. I would do this for three or four laps each time. It must have looked pretty strange to Rose. I remember just suddenly arising from my chair and "walking the circuit."

It seemed to become a ritual, maybe a healing ritual that was just outside of my conscious mind. I did not set a time to walk; I did not look at the clock and tell myself to walk in sixty minutes. My body would simply arise and begin walking; there seemed a sense of urgency about this walking. As I began to walk more and more, the laps became a little faster each time.

Once the "circuit" became too small, I began to walk outside my house; not too far though, just far enough to make a difference. Again, the feelings of vulnerability were omnipresent. What if there was a vicious dog out while I was walking? What if some untoward person decided to mug me as I was walking? These are things that I normally do not think about, but now my personal security mode was in the highest alert.

I live in the middle of a block in my neighborhood; I began walking down the street to the end of the block and back again. I did this for some time. Once, I tried to walk around the whole block, but again, just a few feet away from my usual turn around spot I panicked and went back home. After all, what if

I just ran out of energy on the other side of the street—that would be very awkward and possibly dangerous.

At about the ten-week postoperative period, I began to work my biceps and triceps with my dumbbells. If I were careful, I could isolate these muscle groups without hurting my incision. Again, I could only use one arm—putting the weight in two arms would be too painful on my chest. Rose began to use some workout material she had and we started working out together. Soon after that, I began walking around the block, then the neighborhood, then walking for forty-five minutes three times a week.

I began doing stuff around the house; light housework, some laundry, and began thinking of ways to spend money. Unfortunately, it was around this time that my emotions became very unstable. I do not recall being aware of the severity of these shifting emotions, however, Rose does. She said that I became mostly irritated, mean, and unsatisfied. Additionally, Rose remembers my emotions being unstable or having "emotional lability" in psychobabble from just prior to surgery until we took measures to prevent this at about the fourth month of recovery.

The Emotional Roller-Coaster

It seems that I have intimated throughout this writing that the emotional roller coaster probably started prior to the actual surgical procedure itself. As Rose and I have looked back on that period in our lives, it seems that I began displaying depressive symptoms at least a year prior to the surgery. I had begun to have interpersonal struggles with the people at my place of employment to such a degree that I was discharged on a "medical discharge" from the military organization I was in for "depression." I began to have thoughts that these people were trying to persecute me. Indeed, there is a strong case that what they did was wrong, but I took it more personal than I think was healthy.

I had intense difficulty in falling asleep due to my ruminating over how irritated I was with the way things were going in my life. I had taken a very appealing assignment and began finishing my education in preparation for my career after the military. I thought that the agreement was made between me and the management that I would be at that assignment until my retirement. Therefore, I finished up my bachelor's degree and began work on my master's degree.

Unfortunately, I did not participate in a college savings program when I signed up, and this organization did not typically disperse tuition assistance funding like the other military organizations. Consequently, I shouldered 99.5% of the cost of my education. Therefore, I was not only emotionally invested in my education; I had spent much time and effort over years of my life on this endeavor, along with many thousands of dollars. Unfortunately, the management decided that they wanted me to move to another assignment after they said I could stay there! I was only three months away from graduation! I began to spiral into a deep depression.

I was working full time at the military job, going to school full time, and as part of my education, my practicum was working at a hospice as a marriage and family therapist trainee around 20 hours a week. It was almost more than I could handle, and this hectic pace in varying degrees lasted from 1996 until 1999! I was taking anti-depressant medication and using sleeping pills in order to make it through these tough times. All the while, my heart was beginning to fail. All the while, my brain was being deprived of the optimum amount of nutrients it needed to function most advantageously.

I have been exposed to many of the "positive thinkers" and "faith" people, and other such self-help theories, but quite frankly, none of that worked for me during this time. Surviving open-chest heart surgery is serious business. The pain is excruciating, the way the body is literally sawed open produces discomfort even in the smallest of movements. It takes time for the lungs to clear out the fluids from the bypass machine, so merely breathing is an effort.

The very important coughing is another excruciatingly painful event, and the breathing is difficult. After this description, can you imagine what it was like to sneeze? It takes much, much more than a positive attitude to recover from this optimally.

I address the painful aspects of this surgery to refer to the psychological aspects of the surgery. In other words, my suspicion is that if the person who undergoes this kind of surgery has had previous trauma, it logically follows that they will probably suffer the most psychic wounding around being helpless, the seemingly endless pain, the need to be constantly watched, and other more subtle aspects of the surgery and recovery stage.

In an even more elegant theory, I would suspect that if a person has some genetic predisposition toward "depression" or another "mental disorder" that is interactive with the neurotransmitters in the brain such as Serotonin, Dopamine and other neurotransmitters that are said to play an important role in the mood of a person, then the intensity of this surgery is sufficient to exacerbate this disorder, even if for a short time.

In my particular case, I had been taking Paxil, an antidepressant that is usually used for depressive symptoms that include an anxiety component. Evidently, I was becoming more and more agitated and Rose became very concerned.

I began to try and perform tasks around the house. Rose and I had just bought a new house and we had some ideas of things that we needed to do to make it "our home." We bought a surround sound system, and I actually mounted the little speakers on our ceiling. I used a power drill, but did my hands ever *shake* while performing this task. I then seemed to be driven to do other tasks around the house. I painted the garage, walls, ceilings and floor. I did some gardening things, and suddenly I was spending money like we had it to burn.

Even though I was succeeding in performing these tasks, I became more and more agitated. In the mornings, I would be riding our stationary bicycle as part of my recovery program and would be weeping one minute, then be blazing mad the next. These shifts in mood were dramatic and would happen many times in a day.

As a marriage and family therapist intern, I know that marriages and relationships go through cycles of closeness and distance, trouble and calm, good times and bad throughout their life cycles. Our marriage had seen its struggles just like any other marriage, and things had been particularly difficult the year prior to my surgery. In fact, I had been feeling so guilty that Rose was going to take care of me during my recovery from surgery that I felt compelled to tell her that I had been thinking about getting a divorce, and so maybe we should hire out my care, or she should let me do most of the work. I did not feel right about wanting a divorce and then having her take care of me. Little did I know that someone from the "Mended Hearts" association had told Rose that I might say "some pretty mean things" and that she should "not take them personally." In fact, a colleague of Rose's from work told her that her partner had had bypass surgery and that he left her after the surgery! They eventually got back together.

I was shutting people out of my life left and right. Some of the shutting out was necessary and prudent. For instance, my alcoholic father was so narcissistically injured by my pre surgery letter that just a few days after my coming home from surgery, he got drunk and was harassing Rose and me on the telephone. As is his modus operandi, he is one of those drunks that gets "oiled up" and calls people on the telephone and says awful things to them.

During the early stage of my recovery, the doctors were clear that I was not to have a lot of emotional stress. Therefore, I "fired" him and my mother as parents since they are not safe, and Rose had to contact another family member to get this drunk to stop this behavior.

However, to shut Rose out of my life was a particularly poor decision on my part, and she did not listen to me anyway, for which I will be eternally grateful to her.

Additionally, since I am in the field of therapy, I do like to "walk the walk" as well as "talk the talk." I had been seeing a therapist for over two years. This had been an exceptionally fruitful relationship for me and a real learning experience. We had terminated therapy a few months previous to my surgery in a healthy way. Shortly after my heart surgery, I started back up in therapy. However, shortly after this, I shut my therapist out after a botched attempt at an inpatient treatment facility for "aggravated depression." I was convinced I was having a bipolar reaction due to the severity of my mood swings. My therapist and the intern psychiatrist at the inpatient facility for mood disorders kept saying, "aggravated depression." I did not see this as a valid diagnosis in the Diagnostic and Statistical Manual, Fourth Edition (DSM-IV) (the diagnostic bible for mental health workers) and as mentioned previously, I was convinced that the surgery had exacerbated a heretofore quiet but underlying Bipolar II disorder. I had mentioned to my cardiologist that I was having mood swings and was taking a mood stabilizer and he replied, "Do you really have to take it? Now we will never get the INR levels right!" Obviously, I did not have a sympathetic ear there.

However, I did not stay at the inpatient facility since I was on a voluntary admission. Furthermore, I did not call important friends or colleagues of mine during this time and I began to become paranoid.

At this time, I was terrified of being in a public place and not being able to defend my wife or myself. At some level, this does go back to my own childhood trauma of being held prisoner at the whim of a person bigger and more powerful than myself and being exposed to threats of harm, cursed at, humiliated, shamed and other emotionally abusive behaviors, and there was nothing I could do about it. Nonetheless, I am convinced that a complicated interplay of biopsychosocial dynamics had a significant part to play in the behaviors that I had come to display at that time.

Biologically, I had undergone a severe change in my body chemistry due to the surgery itself. One such change that was confirmed by neuropsychological testing is that my visual memory has been adversely affected by the surgery. Additionally, an EEG revealed a mild slowing of my brain waves in the left temporal lobe of my brain. Temporal lobe damage can also cause emotional lability. Therefore, this psychologist diagnosed me with "mood disorder caused by a general medical condition." I had also gone to a psychiatrist at the behest of my PCP and he diagnosed me with the same condition, only he used old language, "organic mood disorder" from an earlier version of the DSM. This surgery and my psychological reaction to it as noted above served to have a tremendous impact on how the neurotransmitters reacted in their synaptic gaps (essentially the gaps between brain cells) to produce mood lability or "swings," and sociologically I had been "socialized" to expect the worst from certain types of individuals and situations as described by the news, textbooks, and self-discovery.

Additionally, I had come to a resolution in my life that was formed from my childhood experiences that I could trust no one, and that no one could actually take care of me without hurting me. Therefore, being so vulnerable and helpless was intensely difficult for me. One psychiatrist I met who was contracted by the VA to reevaluate me for an increased disability rating was board certified in a number of areas and specialized in Posttraumatic Stress Disorder (PTSD). It was her opinion that my PTSD had also been reactivated by the surgery.

After going to so many health care providers it all became "clear as mud," and I am a therapist! It was not until I began writing this book that my diagnosis seems to be clear. The constant theme is one of a mood disorder due to general medical condition (remember the brain damage in the temporal lobe area?). There is also an underlying depressive and anxiety condition that was already there prior to surgery. And, the posttraumatic stress disorder material began to come back to the surface as a result of the helplessness post surgery. The surgery was the important catalyst that exacerbated all of these conditions. A doctor would say, "Yes, but you are alive!" I agree at this time in my recovery. However, a couple of months after surgery, I would not have agreed with this. In fact, one day after I had gone to work, I began to feel bad physically. I had already come to grips with dying, and so rather than go to the hospital, I just went home, placed linens on the recliner to lie on, and lay there prepared to die.

Pushing Too Hard, Too Fast

I tried to go back to work the third month of recovery although my cardiologist had advised against it. I had become bored with being at home all day, and I did want to begin making money again.

I missed my clients as well. In fact, they were the most enjoyable part about my job. I made an agreement with the clinic manager and my clinic supervisor to see only so many clients and also that I would be attending cardiac rehabilitation at the hospital three days a week in the afternoon.

I work at a county facility, and accordingly it is extremely busy. Much too busy for the small staff that they had and the tension was evident in every staff member's daily routines. I still had a sensitive chest, and could still fatigue easier than before, and I suppose my unit manager did not have time to appreciate this. He kept saying to me, "Whenever you are ready to take more clients and more responsibility, just let me know." I remember feeling harassed. I was still feeling somewhat paranoid and irritated. He pushed me once too hard and I went back to the doctor and took out on a leave of absence for two more months after just two and a half weeks back to work. I remember being absolutely incensed as he was a licensed clinician and I expected more compassion from him.

Rose tells me that I had voiced concerns that this supervisor was "keeping a file on me," more of the paranoid material that frankly I do not remember. At about this time, she was contacting my previous therapist and trying to understand what was happening to me. My therapist advised Rose that she could not talk to her due to confidentiality issues. However, she recommended that Rose call my primary care physician. I received a call from his office to come in. I remember thinking to myself, "it is not a normal occurrence for the doctor's office to call me," and so I called the office.

The receptionist explained, "The doctor just needs to see the patients he has on medication to monitor them, that's all." Normally one has to call in and wait for an appointment for a week or so down the line. This appointment was for that same afternoon.

When I got to the doctor's office Rose was already there. When we were in the office with the doctor she said, "There is something wrong with Rick, his emotions are all out of whack!" The doctor had earned my complete trust, and so I was able to relate to him what I felt was happening. This was when he placed me on a mood stabilizing drug and referred me to a psychiatrist to ensure his diagnosis and medication regimen were appropriate.

It was at this point when I underwent so many of the tests

that I have mentioned previously. The psychiatrist that I saw, who seemed to specialized in geriatric psychiatry, took my information and referred me to have a CT scan. He also recommended that I take a certain powerful new drug in the antipsychotic family called Zyprexa, that works mostly with the Serotonin and dopamine systems in the brain and is helpful for people struggling with organicity problems (physically based problems in the brain that cause mood swings). This drug made me too sleepy, and I eventually found that it affected my INR levels, so the cardiologist had to readjust my dosage. I came off of the drug a couple of weeks later and the INR had to be readjusted again. However, when this psychiatrist read the CT Scan of my brain, he found that the Sulci, or the spaces between brain matter, seemed to be larger than normal, which would be consistent with cerebral atrophy, or the "wasting" of the brain matter.

There are scientific studies that suggest that bypass surgery does indeed produce a degree of cerebral atrophy in some cases. However, for a concrete diagnosis, we would have had to have had a CT Scan of my brain prior to the surgery to compare as a baseline with the post CT Scan.

After the medication that my PCP prescribed to me finally began to reach therapeutic levels in my blood, my mood swings became less and less pronounced. I still experience and continue to experience daily periods of mood lability, but I can use my own cognitive skills to keep them under control. Or in my own theoretic language, I use my observing ego to unhook my emotional wagon to emotionally laden material and this helps me to tolerate the discomfort.

My PCP also referred me for the EEG, which found the mild brain wave slowing in the left temporal lobe area. The neurologist agreed with the doctor's medicine regimen. Yet, the discomfort continued and I ended up going to the VA psychiatry department some time later since my insurance does not cover civilian psychiatrist visits. It was at the VA that I met a resident psychiatrist who I think completed the medicine regimen that has worked the most effectively for me. After she and I talked, she arrived at a provisional diagnosis of Bipolar II and she added a small dose of antidepressant to my mood stabilizer regimen. This seemed to take the severity of the agitation down to a tolerable level. What was interesting about this visit is that she was discussing my case with her supervisor, and they both came up with the Bipolar II disorder, just as I had.

There are no absolutes in psychiatry or psychology and so I am more and more convinced that in cases such as mine, the patient simply must be passionately involved in their own care in order to obtain the best possible outcome.

They must also offer the health care providers as much pertinent information as possible, and they must be *persistent* with their care providers

Once the medication regimen stabilized my mood, I seem to be doing pretty well. I am working and am considering going back to school to pursue a Ph.D. I have contacted most of the people I have known and cared about and resumed a relationship with them. However, I am not the same person I used to be, and I never will be.

Chapter 3

Changed Perspectives

Back from Death

I visited the cardiac surgeon's office for a three-month follow up. One of the PA's who had been on my surgery team was there to conduct this visit. I enjoyed this PA and admired his professionalism, though I never had much of a chance to speak with him directly. He listened to my heart and asked various questions and pronounced me well. I then took the opportunity to ask a few of my own questions.

I asked him what method they used to stop my heart. He replied, "It's much like when they execute a prisoner by lethal injection, we inject a chemical that stops your heart from beating after we anesthetize you." He went on, "We then keep your heart very cold while it is being worked on." I remember saying," so it was like I was dead? He replied, "Yes, clinically dead but being kept alive by a respirator and bypass machine."

I do not know why, but ever since this conversation took place, I have tried to understand the enormity of this operation. It has changed me profoundly, and yet, the magnitude of the process and the ability to articulate my thoughts and feelings about it seems to escape me.

I have read accounts of "near death experiences" where the person journeys into a tunnel or is enveloped in white light. None of this happened in my experience. Yet, I was clinically dead. Now, afterwards, I view many things in my life differently. For instance, I am no longer so fearful of death. I have already been dead, so to speak, and this has taken some of the fear away. At some level, I believe that the spirit lives on and now that I have actually been dead, if I die tomorrow it will be okay with me. This experience took much of the mystery and sting out of death. I have done much of what I have wanted in my life. I also know that my condition can worsen at any time due to blood clotting or thinning complications and I can die at any time and this no longer makes me feel angry or fearful. It does make me sad sometimes, mostly because of how I will miss certain people and things, and that I think Rose will be in pain from the separation my death will cause. This hurts me even now to think of her sadness.

I no longer feel so much self-doubt. At some level, I can now begin to sit with my own decisions and feel reasonably comfortable that they are within my own belief system, social mores, theoretical position, and will not hurt anyone intentionally. This had been a serious struggle for me ever since I can recall. I had always doubted my own intentions, actions, and would suffer tremendous guilt and discomfort after making a decision that affected someone else either positively or negatively. However, after my "death" I seem to have more self-confidence about my decisions. Major life events do not seem to have the level of importance to me that they once did. For instance, if my job fails, I would normally go through an intense depression, get very angry, lose sleep, and feel hopeless. Now, I have been faced with loss of income from being out of work for five months, the possible loss of the brainpower that I once may have had, and the physiologically driven emotional lability, and I can truly say that I deal with these issues much more effectively than I could ever have done before. Oh, I still get emotionally upset and I can feel depressive symptoms approach, but deep within my being I know that nothing short of extreme physical torture at the hands of an enemy can hurt me worse at this point in my life. This is somehow quite freeing.

Embracing Limitations

My cardiac surgeon told me after the surgery that "you will be as good as new in six months." Well, I do look pretty good at the six-month period. My incision still hurts a little at times, and I can swear that there is an annoying tingling sensation where the wire was used to tie my chest bones together. But then the surgeon modified his previous statement after the surgery and told me when I asked if I would be able to resume my love of weight lifting, "You can use light weights, but the valve is not designed for heavy weights—it can't handle the pressure."

For whatever reason, I only "heard" a part of this, and as soon as the fourth month, I began to do some heavier weight lifting. I seemed able to do it as long as I was not working and took a nap during the day. However, I have found at the sixth month that I cannot handle doing heavy weights while working full time. I have modified my lifting to lighter weights and more repetitions. Initially, this made me a little sad, but it is another grief and loss issue of losing the self that I once was. This seems to be working pretty well for me. Of course, it always helps the motivational levels to have a workout partner, and my wife is mine.

Another limitation is extreme changes in temperature. I have loved to keep my own lawn, and during my military career my lawns were recognized by the organizations as being very good and good for the organization's image. My new house has a wonderful lawn and I was very much enjoying keeping it manicured. It was a different kind of grass that I was used to dealing with and it is very beautiful when manicured properly. However, I live in the San Joaquin Valley where the summer temperatures exceed 100 degrees regularly. Rose noticed that after I would do the lawn on Saturday, I would not be able to recover from this for two days, sleeping in late on Sunday and not being able to do our workouts on Monday. We hypothesized that it was the work on the lawn in the heated conditions that took its toll on my body. We recently hired the lawn care out to a professional service. Another loss issue.

I used to be fairly organized in my thinking processes, and now I tend to find myself "forgetting" what I was just trying to say. Another loss issue.

Loss is an issue that I can deal with more easily ever since my surgery. Prior to my surgery I was operating from the traumatized part of my being that was taught that I was defective just by "being." I now know that I have a genuine heart condition and connected organic mood disorder and somehow this has freed me from thinking it has always been me being a defective soul.

Retraining

Some heart patients who had previously stressful jobs or jobs that involved heavy physical work might have to retrain themselves for another career. My surgeon assured me that I would be "good as new within six months after the surgery." In fact, I am doing quite well; however, I do have some physical limitations that Rose has begun to bring to my attention.

I am not able to do physical labor in moderate to severe heat. Rose started noticing that it took me two, sometimes three days of rest to recover from yard work or trying to wash my motor home. This is so different from what I was capable of before the surgery. I am unable to have a day that is packed full of activities. For instance, I cannot perform housework, work an eight-hour day, and do my cardiovascular workouts all in the same day. I have always been very physical and can no longer express that part of myself. At this point in my recovery I get up and exercise at 4:00 a.m., work an eight-hour day and by then I am fairly tired.

If your career is in a heavy labor field, there are usually state-funded programs that will retrain you for another job. Of course, I heartily recommend college or vocational schools for anyone because these institutions seem to provide the most solid chances for employment after all the effort and cost that is put in the retraining. Additionally, the starting wage of a college graduate or technical school graduate is generally higher. There is also financial aid at most colleges and universities that can help with living costs.

Chapter 4

A Desire for Dialogue With the Medical, Psychological and Spiritual Professionals

Freedom of Choice

One subject that I am reticent to mention due to its highly controversial nature is the notion of freedom of choice for the patient in deciding if they desire to have the surgery or not, as well as having an active input into their care. My perspective has come full circle on this issue since my surgery.

My experience working with the hospice as a bereavement volunteer and marriage and family therapist trainee was a poignant and powerful experience for me. It allowed me a chance to view death close up and personal. I had to confront my own fears about the death process, my own reaction to it, and my being able to experience the reactions of others who are experiencing the death of a loved one in a way that is respectful and thoughtful to the healing process.

The hospice nurses who trained the bereavement volunteers were extremely knowledgeable, compassionate and tenaciously dedicated to their work. They taught us in modules with didactic information and shared their personal experiences with us. I remember vividly the day they explained pain management for the dying. It was very straightforward: there is a subjective scale from 1 to 10, 1 being almost asleep but relatively free from the intensity of the pain, and 10 being in excruciating pain. The patient was to have the freedom of choice to decide at what times of the day they would be relatively pain free or more "awake" for visiting with their family members. The nurses also explained that to their knowledge at the time, which was 1999, the mainline doctor course load provided one basic seminar on pain management. Therefore, doctors are not by any stretch of the imagination, "experts" in the field of pain management. They explained that the doctor running the hospice had taken numerous courses and conducted his own study of pain management and therefore it was concluded in this particular hospice that no patient was to suffer from their pain. Their pain was to be managed effectively through close consultation with the doctor.

The hospice patients were receiving what is called "palliative" care. In other words, no aggressive effort was being made to heal their sickness or disease since these were considered beyond amelioration and a prognosis of death within a year was given. However, a very loving and competent effort was being made to help these patients die with dignity and respect. Living in their own homes, they would be bathed, given a bed that would be safe for them if they needed it, helped with medication by the professional staff, and volunteers would be available for help with grocery shopping or reading stories or babysitting for caregivers who need to "get out for a while."

In my opinion, our society has denied death by institutionalizing it to such a point that we as a nation no longer wish to see it. We would prefer to send our sick and dying to the hospital and let them die there in a clean, sterile environment tended to by unknown professionals and volunteers. This way, we do not have to deal with the emotional material that is stirred up in us as a result of watching someone dying.

Contrariwise, the hospitals seem to be in denial about the humanity of the patient. It seems as if the doctors and nurses in the hospital setting say to themselves, "We cannot let the patient voice negative statements about their health, nor can I give them any minute cause for concern or this might negatively affect the outcome of the treatment process." Additionally, they must build up a protective wall around their own humanity due to the horrendous sights and deeply emotional events that they see on an almost daily basis. The patient of course would see this as the staff being somewhat distant and cold.

Some doctors and nurses hold to the "placebo effect" when talking to patients. The classic example of this is where the physician gives a patient a "sugar pill" for specific symptoms the patient is describing, and tells the patient that this powerful drug will have them feeling better in no time. The data reveal that this can work and in some cases can work in almost 45 to 50 percent of the cases in a certain study. I have reviewed various scholarly articles on this subject and while there are data to support the importance of this clinical tool, I eschew its use due to the dishonest nature at the base of its conception. I am passionately dedicated to honesty in the health care profession.

When I was told that I had to undergo surgery, at some level I knew that I had the choice to say "no." However, Rose and I talked about it, and she was so respectful, she let me make the decision. I decided on the surgery. The doctors did not address the idea of having an option. Instead, it seemed that their protocol was based upon going into the patient's room and encouraging them to have the surgery and that "everything would be just fine." Using some of the placebo effect along with some neurolinguistic programming "start speaking what you want to happen" and smart sales techniques because, after all, they do want the business. Moreover, "people want to go to doctors that know everything and have the confidence that they will heal them." I suspect that our society is a bit more sophisticated than that at this stage in our cultural developmental process. I am not sitting in moral judgment on this issue, instead I am addressing as many of the salient issues involved in making a decision for surgery as I can.

I now know that at this point in my life, if I had to have another open-chest heart surgery I would choose not to have it. It is just too painful and financially destructive to my life and the lives of my family. However, I was discussing this issue with my friend and mentor, Dr. Dennis Wong, and it seemed from our brief conversation about this issue that he felt that the decision not to have the surgery could also be self-centered on my part and I could be thinking *for* my family instead of *respecting* their desires. This was part of a larger conversation about the bioethics of heart surgery, a subject that he advised against my tackling in my doctoral work due to the enormity of the subject and the need for a realistic timeframe to complete my other work. I thought about that very deeply for some time and decided that indeed, if a person is in a long-term relationship with another person, or is the parent of a child, that person must be respectful enough of the other person to enter into an open dialogue concerning the upcoming life or death decision. The patient must include them somehow in their thought processes, and also elicit the feelings and thoughts of the other person. I will say from my own experience that I was definitely in a state of shock at the time that Rose and I had to discuss the issue, and she was in just as much shock, maybe even more and I know that this hindered a complete discussion for both of us. She is older than I am and she always kind of thought that she would be the first to have these kinds of problems. We discussed the issues in "units of work" or small discreet conversations that we could tolerate in our effort to arrive at a final decision about the surgery.

However, as I write this work, I still fall back to my original position that ultimately the person must always have the right to choose for him or herself, no matter what others may say. I simply must have the right to choose if I want the surgery, and

I must also have the right to choose not to have the surgery. The patient must also have the right to have adequate pain management, regardless of whether or not it makes them "sleepy." I am still quite angry about the way that my pain management was handled while I was in the hospital. I recall literally begging for Demerol, which works very well for me, but I was told that it makes me sleep and this would not let me heal properly. Well, I maintain that I could have performed my walking and coughing in the morning, and toward the afternoon when I was trying to sleep; I could have had some Demerol to ease the excruciating pain. Then toward the evening, I could have done more rehabilitative work.

Imagine the barbarity of sawing a person's chest open, and then only giving them enough pain medication to "take the edge off." This seems frighteningly similar to what a sadist would do when torturing someone. If they are worried about addiction, this is an issue that should be addressed post treatment. I have treated addictions for a number of years in a treatment center, and not only in my opinion, but in the opinion of many properly licensed treatment professionals that addicts must receive pain medication when warranted, and then get right back on their recovery from addictions program afterwards. To do otherwise is truly brutal and primitive and reminds me of when I read about the Nazi atrocities where certain "doctors" performed surgery on un-anesthetized Jews.

If failure to provide adequate pain medication for open-chest heart surgery patients is an insurance issue, then we must push for reforms in this system. As my mentor Dr. Wong reminded me, our generation is the largest generation yet, and we are getting older. Our generation is going to start having these heart conditions in record numbers and while we have the technological prowess to deal quite effectively with this dynamic, I suppose that the insurance companies might begin "denying" adequate medication for pain.

Granted, each individual has their own unique threshold for pain tolerance, which essentially disputes the theory that people do not heal properly when medicated with pain medications since all of us are different. And since there is no way that they can measure the subjectiveness of pain tolerance and treatment outcomes due to the subjective scales simply not being reliable enough to be measured accurately in a scholarly study; therefore, a reputable study could not effectively use a "universal amount of medication" for a certain surgical condition and come up with the "correct" amount. Furthermore, each person reacts differently to medication. I received a wonderfully helpful package from the American Heart Association. It contained a brochure about valve replacement surgery and explained: "pain medication should will be given liberally for the first few days…" I still shudder at how mine was withheld. If you are going to undergo open-chest heart surgery, insure that you have a frank chat with your cardiac surgeon about pain management.

Thus, my desired dialogue with the medical community is to challenge them to challenge their own "beliefs" about pain management as well as what their own thoughts and beliefs are about death, dying and the healing process. Questions that I strongly desire the medical health care providers to ask themselves are: "Do I believe in telling the patient the truth, no matter what the material is?" "Why am I in this field, is it for the money?" "Do I believe that healing is a process that only has room for 'positive thinking' and denial of 'negative thinking' to the point of denying the patient the right to voice their own truth?" "Am I burned out enough that I need to find a different line of work?" "Am I doing the job in this field that I have always wanted to do?" "Why not?" "Do I find it a joy to work with patients?" "Does life have a certain sacredness to me?" "Am I afraid of death?" "Am I afraid of my own feelings?" "Do I dread talking to the families of the patients?" These are deeply probing questions and each of these questions should stir up a great deal of material in the health care professional that asks them seriously of themselves.

Does the Left Hand Know What the Right Hand is Doing?

Another conversation with my mentor gave me pause to think: there is a split between the medical and the psychological communities. One community thinks of the person as an elegant amalgam of exquisitely complex systems. The other community treats the person as an incredibly complex supernatural being that cannot be totally explained by the systems that encompass them.

In my exposure to the Eastern schools of medicine, the body and soul or life essence are wonderfully intertwined and what impacts one part or piece of the human being, impacts the other, much like the Western field of psychoneuroimmunology is beginning to recognize. For instance, it is now commonly known that stress produces an abundance of chemicals such as corticosteroids to name one, in the body that begins to "break down" its immune system. Thus, we have an energy force such as human interaction producing an effect on the physical body. It is also common knowledge that stress raises the blood pressure in humans; therefore, certain stress reducing exercises are given to counteract this dilemma, such as deep breathing, visualization, and sometimes medication for the more serious conditions.

It is not my intention in this current work to point out the concrete differences between all eastern and western views on the mind-body concepts and healing. I will be addressing some of this in another work in the next couple of years. However, in this country it has been known for some time that there is an incredible difference in how the Western medical, psychological and spiritual communities are segregated. Slowly, there is a growing movement to eliminate this split, but in my experience, it seems to be moving at a snail's pace. Somehow, I would suspect that politically with respect to licensure to practice issues, and insurance issues with regard to how much and to who is paid for what, is the slowing force in keeping the split between medicine, psychology, and spirituality apart.

In review concerning the baby boomer generation being bigger than any generation and getting older, it strikes me that all three of the areas mentioned above need to reassess their views on death and dying. In a story from my own family, my grandmother was a devout religious woman who attended church every Sunday faithfully unless sick. She had been in a situation where her kidneys were shutting down and it was painful for her to keep living. Her pastor reportedly came into the room to visit and instead of simply providing the spiritual care that was confident of the after-life, he would not let anyone say that she might die. In fact, the prayer was that she not be "taken home yet." This for a number of reasons alarms me; specifically, as is a theme throughout my book, the patient was not asked what she wanted, it was assumed for her. Moreover, that particular belief system teaches a wonderful place for the person's spirit or soul to reside when one's body dies, and it is supposed to be a very important and awesome moment for the person when they die. Not to deny the sadness of the separations and the tears of grief by everyone concerned, but to deny the very belief system by the recognized oracle of the belief system is incongruent and confusing for all three areas that are split. The psychologists then begin to criticize the clerics, and vice versa, and then the doctors just want all of these people out of the way so that they can "treat the patient."

It should be noted at this point that I am an advocate for patient rights and choice for adults. I am also an advocate for children to have this right within reason. If a child has a deadly disease and the treatments are very painful, they should have the option of not taking the treatment with or without parental consent. For instance, there should be a vehicle in place that if a young child has already had a heart transplant and needs another one, they should be able to refuse the treatment, even if the parents push for it.

There is the argument that if I choose not to have another surgery on my heart and I need it, but am suffering from depressive symptoms that I am not in a lucid state of mind to make that decision for myself. However, I would argue that only when it can be ascertained that I am in a "deep" part of the depression or a psychosis that my opinion would not be well-informed. Once again, this is tricky, because it is all very subjective and ultimately the patient must endure the pain and suffering of the surgical and recovery procedures.

To Have or Not to Have

Now that I have had my surgery, I can look back and see how it has affected my own psychological well-being, my wife's psychological well-being, my finances, and my outlook on the future.

It is possible that I have a rather morbid view of certain aspects of the life cycle process, but in a way, I am glad that I had the surgery and that it saved my life, and I am also not so glad that it happened. I am glad to be alive because I am having a lot more fun than I used to, and my mood is much better for the most part and this is probably due to the mood stabilizers that I am on.

However, I was out of work for over five months and I understand that I am lucky to have had a job to come back to, as some employers do not hold jobs open for long medical leaves of absences. If I had not received a lump sum payment from the military organization that I was in prior to my surgery I would have dragged my wife and I into bankruptcy court. My insurance covered all $80,000 (approximate) of the surgery, but

I still needed to pay my bills, and I was only receiving a very small sum from the state disability. I could envision going bankrupt and trying to keep the house while Rose was working and us trying to eat and keep the creditors away until the bankruptcy process took over. What an awful thought. When, conversely, I have a life insurance policy that would have made things much more comfortable for Rose if I would have died.

I recall a client coming into my office who had been a worker all of his life, just not in one place, and had only recently begun recovering from bypass surgery. He came to see me because he was depressed due to his state disability check having been stopped and he was not able to get federal disability yet as this process takes many months, and he and his partner were not able to make ends meet. He was spiraling into a deep depression. His physical body was repaired, but his emotional well-being was a casualty of the surgical and other environmental processes. I was not able to continue with this client due to my having to go back out on a leave of absence of my own; I only pray that he made progress in his journey.

I also remember hearing some of the retired survivors talking about how they had to take out loans to pay for their surgeries. However, since they were on a fixed income before, their finances were not so disastrously affected. Notwithstanding, I was made aware of an older couple that did not have insurance and they somehow were "blessed" with someone paying the surgical bills, but they cannot afford the medication. Therefore, they drive from Washington State all the way down to Mexico to get this person their heart medications.

I guess what I am speaking of is quality of life issues post surgery. I think that this should be an important factor in how one makes the decision to have the surgery or not to have it. What will it cost me in terms of physical limitations, financial hardships, relational difficulties, and general healthiness? What will it benefit me in terms of things that I feel I have left unfinished, or how will it benefit my family or others? Just because we have the technology to fix a physical problem, should we? Just because we can replace someone's heart, lung, or kidney, should we? Are we as a society ready to help those of us who are trying to recover from surgery via government programs, or are we as a society just going to piously say, "Of course a person should *always* be allowed surgery" without providing a source of disability income to help them. If our government is unwilling to set aside funding for such personal disasters, can "faith-based support groups" take up the slack. In my experience, they cannot.

Just prior to my surgery when President Clinton was in office, there was a huge surplus of dollars and it appeared to some "experts" that social security was going to be "saved" or at least given a fighting chance to stay solvent. However, at the time of this writing, it seems that social security will now not be able to pay all of the members who have contributed to it starting in the next few years. Instead, we are advised to personally invest in the stock market to cover our retirement costs. My question is what about the people who are disabled. I was not sure that I would be able to go back to my job or work at all due to my mood instability. Therefore, I applied to the Social Security Insurance program to get a "head start on the paperwork." My experience with them was very negative. Even though I paid into this system for over *30 years*, I was initially denied benefits because I was receiving a small amount from the state and I did not meet their criteria for "permanently" disabled even though the SSI program is touted as a "back-to-work program." It has been months since I applied, and so far, I have only been psychologically tested to ascertain the degree of brain damage that I incurred from the surgery and that is all. In fact, when I spoke with the disability evaluator she pretty much intimated to me that I would not be qualified for SSI even during my recovery when I could not work.

My dialogue with the medical, psychological, and spiritual community on this issue is this: why are we pushing and striving for such amazing technology and for all people to use this technology when we as a nation do not help these same people keep from ending up in poverty?

I am reminded of a client of mine who had a mechanical heart valve. I had been treating him for addiction issues and he was generally responding to the treatment provided. Later, after my own experience with heart surgery and my own review of the scholarly literature, this person's mental illness diagnoses, and the psychological effects of heart surgery on patients after the surgery, I am convinced that this is a missing element in his treatment process. He had a house, family, and a good job. However, now he lives as a homeless man, pretty much out of contact with his family, who comes to county mental health for his treatments: do we do this all for the sake of tenaciously hanging onto any shred of life we can have? Can we really call living homeless and destitute "life?" An argument might be made that he is choosing to live that way. I would also argue that if he could have been provided financial assistance during a recovery phase, things might be radically different in his life. Yet these are basically secular issues, there are many different views on this same subject with regard to spirituality. However, I am speaking strictly in the secular sense for the purpose of addressing the financial aspects of the recovery period since money tends to shape the environmental elements of the recovery as well.

Again, since the baby boomer generation is aging, these issues concerning recovery after major surgery need to be addressed adequately in the coming years or there will be uninformed decisions being made by patients and health care professionals with tragic consequences. The dilemma of whether the ubiquitous "State" should regulate who gets surgery or not, or who should qualify for financial assistance in the form of welfare, SSI or other such programs or not, or should only the rich get access to the newer technology, has been a constant philosophical debate for as many years as I can remember.

What about our elected officials such as the Vice President? Should he be allowed to serve in office with a malfunctioning heart? The literature is quite clear that certain psychological issues, such as depressive symptoms can occur after heart surgery and can be problematic for years. If military organizations eschew its members from taking psychotropic medication, and most certainly the person under psychological care for "depression" would not be able to handle nuclear weapons, how can the Vice President, a potential commander of our nuclear weapons arsenal, be excused from the rules? What kind of a statement is he making for the rest of the heart patients in the world? It seems to me that at one level he is saying, "Don't be discouraged, you can do whatever you want to do, even with a heart problem." At another level he seems to be stating, "If heart patients are not out working as before in ultra-stressful jobs, they are wimps." Yet, not even into the first year of his term, this man has had at least one heart procedure to stint a coronary artery and one procedure to attach a mechanical device that will "help the doctors monitor his condition."

Could it be that the nation is in denial about heart disease on the micro level, and death and dying issues on the macro level? Does our "marketplace philosophy" so drive our national ideals that we deny the existence of those who are not able to compete, those who are starving in the streets right here in our nation. How can we be congruent with our pious attitudes that say one thing, but our actions say another?

Chapter 5

Having Your Affairs in Order

How Much Trauma Do You Want?
   If you have a heart condition that is allowing you to take time to make informed decisions, or you have a chronic heart condition which poses imminent death in the near future, it would benefit you to think about things in many different areas of your life.
   As a starting place in no particular order of precedence, you should provide the hospital, doctor(s) and other health care professionals with a document that specifically states what kind of "heroics" you wish them to perform on you in case you begin to die. One kind of document that I had was a "living will" which specifically stated that if I had a medical condition that would end in my death in a relatively short time, or leave me in a vegetative state, and the diagnosis was agreed upon by two doctors, all life support measures would be withdrawn to include: cardiopulmonary resuscitation, artificial feeding, artificial hydrating, surgery or any other life-sustaining procedure. I had a military lawyer draw this up for Rose and me prior to my discharge, and it was one of the most important things that I have ever done. It was one less hassle that I had to worry about when my heart valve was going bad; the admission staff asked us, "Do you have any advance directives?" We were able to produce them without any extra effort. There are other legal issues involved such as, limited or full powers of attorney to your spouse or a relative or a friend that you can trust, as well as your last will and testament. These are all incredibly

important issues to have resolved before your surgery if you can.

If you are anything like most of the people that I have come into contact with in my practice of therapy, you are going to be feeling so many different feelings. You will probably be wanting desperately to speak to different people in your life and you will want to talk about your condition with them. It may be easy with some of these people; it might be harder with others. One of my soapbox items is that in my experience and opinion, we are not taught to communicate very effectively by our institutions or our parents. The why is beyond the scope of this book, it just seems to be so. An excellent work on the subject is from Robert! Bolton (1976) in his book, *People Skills*. In it he states, "I have become increasingly aware of the inadequacy of most communication. In our society it is rare for persons to share what really matters—the tender, shy, reluctant feelings, the sensitive, fragile, intense disclosures. It is equally rare for persons to listen intently enough to really understand what another is saying."

Therefore, some people may be more interested in what they are thinking than they are about listening to you, and here you are needing support and they cannot provide that for you. I encourage you not to take it personally and to say what it is you need to say to them—this heart condition is real, and serious, you may only get one chance at this closure thing, take the chance.

Closure is the process of acknowledging the relationship you have had with someone and talking about it. It may sound chic or passé, but, in my opinion, whenever two human beings have interacted with each other and have become involved at least in a semi-intimate way, such as family members, close friends, treasured colleagues, mentors, etc., when it is time to no longer see this person, an improper closure can leave an open wound or mini trauma, if you will in the psyche. In our day and age, we say, "see you later" or "so long." However, this seems to speak volumes of how we as a society only want things "quick and dirty." I have spoken with many clients who have been grieving the loss of a loved one and a constant theme from these folks is that they wished there could have been more of a "goodbye." How sad it is for them to have been deprived of the last few comforting words such as, "I love you honey" or "I'll miss you." I recall one colleague saying that when he visits a home with a dying member, and the family is there, he begins a reminiscence session. What a wonderful idea! Get the family talking about their history, precious moments as well as the foibles; dying is a part of life! This colleague of mine wept as he relayed how one family just had a beautifully healing hour of this kind of communication.

Embrace and revel in the conversations that are soothing to you prior to your surgery, let them linger in your memory and be a comfort to you. Additionally, if you are not finding relief in talking with the people in your sphere of contacts, such as family, friends, or colleagues, then find a competent therapist to talk to. Preferably a therapist with a hospice background or that is comfortable with death and dying issues or a trained pastoral counselor who is comfortable with death and dying issues and will not make you deny your dying process in the name of faith.

On a personal note, prior to my surgery I began to feel extremely needful of clarifying my own spiritual belief system and being congruent with that system. This provided me with some anxiety as in many cases not all folks involved in a spiritual journey are congruent in their journey all the time, just as I was not. I felt a steady drive to connect with my view of God in the most serious way that I have ever done. For some reason, I did not seek out the religious leaders of my faith; instead, I read and did much praying. It was God that I wanted to talk with about spirituality, not human beings. I had no special epiphany before, during, or after the surgery, however, as I mentioned previously in this work; I no longer fear death as I once did. I came to a place where I believe what my spiritual belief system says about my spirit after the death of the physical body and came to embrace this belief. Hal Lindsey writes in his book, *The Late Great Planet Earth* (1970), "...There are no atheists in fox holes...." I suppose that that statement is true for me. Just as the alcoholic or drug addict cannot battle their disease of addiction alone and need a "higher power" to help them in their recovery, so do, I think, people who are facing life and death surgery. This God, higher power, or whatever your belief system is, should be big enough to control the outcome of the surgery and to keep your family safe in the event you are to be taken home to be with Him. To live without this hope seems to leave the person with an anxious fear and dread of the unknown. What a lonely and horrible way to end your life.

Have you and your spouse, family, or partner decided on how you wish your body to be put away in the event of your death? These are also decisions that should be decided prior to your surgery in order not to leave it all to someone else. You may have religious beliefs that have specific instructions about how your body should be handled. Alternatively, you may have a generation of family tradition on this matter. My wife and I have decided that rather than pay the exorbitant prices of caskets and other costs that go along with preparing the body for a viewing, etc., that we will both be cremated after our deaths. This is mostly an issue of cost effectiveness for us. Also, there is one special thing that both of us have promised to do for each other, we have each decided on our favorite places in this country and have asked that our ashes be spread somewhere in these areas.

Chapter 6

Preparing Your Family

Can You Really Talk About What is Happening?
Once you have received the diagnosis, it is time to tell your spouse, or partner, and your children if you have any about your illness. I recall the first day I received the news that I had "moderate to severe aortic valve regurgitation" and would have to be monitored very closely for the rest of my life. My doctor gave me a lot of samples of the "vasodilator" medicine recommended by the cardiologist; a prescription for Clonazepam and off I went to go home. As I was driving to the pharmacy, I recall being in total shock. I remember thinking, "What will Rose say?" "How will she deal with this news?"

> **Clonazepam** or Klonopin is a benzodiazepine anticonvulsant drug that can be effective in "calming" a person down. It is also highly addictive.

When I got home, I remember telling her that the appointment did not go as I expected. Then almost immediately, as always during times of stress, our dysfunctional relational "scripts" or "roles" came right into action. Like some helpless child I blurted out, "I have a bad aortic valve and it is leaking really bad, I have to be on this medication and I have to go in for an echocardiogram every three months!" This script is the "hurt child" and is dysfunctional because I am expecting Rose to take care of me but do not like it when she does. Rose's script or role is the "critical parent" and this comes out because she does not want to take care of a grown child. The dynamic is somewhat more complicated that this, but this is essentially the gist of the transactional analysis theory in our relationship.

Rose replied by literally grilling me with difficult questions about my condition and I was further exasperated by not knowing the answers to these questions. I swear she should have been an interrogator for the military! But we got through it. In the course of some very tough years and dogged effort, we have learned to get through the disfunction and began to communicate effectively in those moments. The dark, dank, overwhelming cloud of feelings hung in the air that night as we pondered the meaning of this new health development for me and what it meant to our relationship. I withdrew and became silent. Rose cried.

I started on the medication and Rose began to become ever watchful over me. For some reason I remember thinking that I was sad that I would have to be on blood pressure medication, but did not think that anything really bad was happening. I was in denial. My doctor's reaction should have told me. However, the cardiologist I have who has just an awful bedside manner did not emphasize anything, he just said that my condition "was serious and would need to be watched closely for the rest of my life." I suspect that Rose had a lesser level of denial than I had. Although I was not actually saying, "Nothing is wrong with me." I just did not seem to grasp the seriousness of the situation.

I do not remember talking very much about this with Rose. I remember being furious at the VA and the military organization I was in because they did not catch this issue that I was sure, and several doctors agreed with me, had to have been quite obvious when I was being checked out of their system. This was not a condition that cropped up in the couple of months that I had been out. It had existed for years. Possibly I began to take my unconscious anger at my having a sick heart out on the VA and the military organization by writing several rather heated letters to request action be taken on my behalf due to this egregious error that had taken place. Those were dark days for Rose and me. And my suspicion is that I am not the only person in America or the world that has been affected by their heart disease in this manner.

Rose and I did not really speak about the gravity of my heart condition until after the angiogram had confirmed my need for immediate surgery. I suppose looking back; I wish that I had been more respectful of our relationship in this area. I was online checking out anything I could about open-heart surgery. There were a couple of good sites that related a very small part of the actual process. More often than not, I basically had to visit several sites that handled small parts of the same subject. However, no data on "living with heart disease" except these little blurbs from the AHA. I wanted to find something that was written by someone who could relate the "personal" aspects of the process like Kottler (1991) did for therapists in his wonderful work, *The Compleat Therapist*. At that time, I could not find anything like this for heart diseases online or in the bookstores.

Time to Say What You Feel

I know now what I will do if my heart condition worsens to the point that death is imminent. I will try my absolute best to spend every spare moment I have with my life partner and take her to places where we like to go. We have this thing for Disneyland, so we would go there at least once or twice before I became too ill to travel. And we would spend a lot of time in the mountains; we are mountain people and love it up there. I would also try to visit my grown children at least once or twice before I got too ill to travel. I would reminisce with them and say goodbye to them. I would pray a lot. And I would spend time looking at this wondrous creation called the Earth and the outdoors, even if it's only from my backyard looking at the sky.

I would go with Rose to pick out my urn, and tell her what clothes I would like to be cremated in. And I would want to spend time telling her either via letter or conversation how important she has been to me in our seventeen years together before any pain or sudden death could interfere with the process. Sudden death is a major concern with heart disease so I would want to do this quickly (I have already done this!).

I would also ask for hospice service if I have been given notice that I was terminally ill. In some states, a person must be diagnosed as going to die within a year to qualify for hospice service. Nevertheless, this would help take much of the pressure of caring for me off Rose and into the hands of competent people who are truly dedicated to ensuring their patients experience "death with dignity." Part of that dignity is to die at home. In my experience, if they would have said, "Rick, the operation did not take and you're going to die if we don't do this…this…or this…" I would have had Rose arrange for ambulance transportation to my house to die.

However, surprisingly, Rose and I were in such shock, we did not take the time to look back and do what I call a "life's review" process. In my practice of therapy, I do this for folks who are dying. This can be elderly people who have had a long life, or this could be someone who is younger and has a terminal illness. Essentially, a life review is a process where one looks back and remembers the good and the bad in a slow and honest fashion. This can take a person to a profound place of enlightenment and contentment. It will bring up many different feelings, and being able to "sit with" those feelings during this review can be very healing. Incidentally, Rose and I have spent many hours doing this review ever since my moods were able to become more stable. What a joy this is! I also have done this life review for my own experiences outside the context of my relationship with Rose. It is my opinion that performing the life review and talking about the "difficult things inside" or taking care of "unfinished business" is two things that seem really important to me looking back on my experience. Something prospective heart surgery patients would do well to consider for themselves.

Chapter 7

A Partner's Perspective

Heart Disease

Heart disease and surgery not only affect the patient; the process also affects their family, friends, and co-workers. My perspective of the year before diagnosis, surgery, and recovery varies in areas from Rick's. As Rick mentioned, open-chest heart surgery is a result of progressive heart disease, not a condition developed over a few days or weeks. Unfortunately, the military doctors in charge of his healthcare did not care enough about their patient to go that extra step in ordering an echocardiogram, disregarding Rick's request to explore his heart murmur.

Looking back over the year before diagnosis, the symptoms should have been obvious to healthcare professionals. He presented with shortness of breath, irritability, depression, running out of energy, and not being able to do his usual workout routine of weight lifting and running. The military healthcare system diagnosed him as having asthma and did recognize depression and anxiety. He also had problems sleeping, needing to sleep longer hours at night with frequent awakenings, and taking 2-3 hour naps during the day. The military doctors tested for sleep apnea, which was inconclusive. Other medical conditions were not investigated. Medical care was limited to giving him pills for anxiety, depression, sleeping and some inhalers for his asthma and sending him out for regular duty. Of course he was not able to perform exceptionally as he had in the past, causing questions about his ability to perform to standards required to be deployed worldwide at any minute. His health condition also caused scrutiny from co-workers and supervisors. Was he faking illness? Was he trying to "work the system"? These accusations actually did occur. They affected Rick personally and professionally, which affected our relationship and his relationship with our daughter. Rick grew increasingly insecure about himself. I thank God that he had the option to accept a medical discharge from the military with a lump sum disbursement instead of a small, monthly retirement check. If he had attempted to stay in the military, he would have died by the end of the year from undiagnosed congestive heart failure.

The Echocardiogram

After the medical discharge, Rick accepted employment with a county agency that provided medical coverage. As soon as medical coverage was in effect, he requested that his primary care physician refer him for an echo. I did not accompany Rick for the echo procedure or the follow-up appointment with his doctor for test results. After all, didn't the military doctors say the heart murmur was nothing to be concerned about? That follow-up appointment confirmed our suspicions that something was indeed wrong with Rick. We just weren't expecting the enormity of the situation. His doctor told him that he had heart disease and would probably require heart surgery in the near future, but at this time would need to be monitored every three months. We were shocked. Rick had always been healthy and worked out. How could this be?

We decided to tell our families. Our son and daughter were shocked. They always thought of Rick as a big, strong, healthy man. My mom and sisters were very sympathetic and shocked as well. I was very angry at the response we received from Rick's family. His mom told him to get a second opinion and his dad said, "You always did have bad luck." One sister sent a card that said, "A forgiving heart is a healed heart." His eldest sister was the only one that showed any compassion at all. I don't remember hearing at all from his youngest sister.

Symptoms quickly escalated. There were times that Rick would go to work, come home, eat and go to bed. He was no longer enthusiastic about working out or running. In fact, he stopped these activities. Rick worked out as often as possible, even while we were dating so this sent up a red flag. We did go camping over a holiday weekend, but I could tell that Rick just didn't have the energy to enjoy himself. Weekends became sleep marathons. One Saturday, Rick went target shooting, one of his passions. We had plans for the evening so he decided to take a little nap because he was tired. I could not get Rick to wake up, much less get him out of bed and to the event. He asked that I go alone since I was on the committee and enjoy myself, and that he would try to make it for dinner. I kept calling home to check on him and found him sleeping each time. He did make it for dinner, but was not able to stay for more than an hour. I went home to find him in bed. He had problems waking and staying up the next day and arose from a nap short of breath. He called the cardiologist and was told to schedule an angiogram for the following week. This time I did accompany Rick for the test and have been with him for every doctor appointment since that date.

The angiogram was done on an outpatient basis. I was allowed to wait with Rick until he was called down to the operating room where the angiograms were performed. During our wait, Rick was given a sedative. It did not affect him very much. He was very anxious. I had to go in search of a medical assistant for a blanket because Rick was cold. I strongly urge that someone be with the patient whenever possible to see that their needs are met. The healthcare system has had such a reduction in staff that patient care has been seriously compromised. I was not allowed to accompany Rick during the procedure. A staff person came up to me in the waiting room and told me the doctor wanted to talk to me; the procedure had been completed. The cardiologist asked me to sit next to him and he began to show me the pictures taken of Rick's heart. He explained, in terms I could understand, what I was looking at. I was amazed that so much blood was gushing in the wrong direction. This statement will be emblazoned in my memory forever: "He is not going to die today, but he will need surgery by the end of this week. We are looking for a bed for him tonight, but if one can't be found, he can come back tomorrow afternoon for surgery on Thursday. We are paging the heart surgeon now." I can remember that statement and play it repeatedly in my mind. I asked if he had told Rick, and he replied, "No, you and Mr. Froyd have a lot to talk about." Then hearing the conversation taking place where Rick was, he called around the corner, "Give Mr. Froyd more Valium, he is a little nervous." The cardiologist told me I could go talk to Rick. Everything around me was blurred. Just recalling the incident brings tears to my eyes. I stood up and the floor seemed inches from my face. I was afraid I was going to faint. How was I going to tell Rick? What if he died during the night? What was I going to do? I entered the operating room and smelled his blood, his life. I walked up to him and relayed word for word what the cardiologist had said. Rick's eyes grew huge and he tried to lift his head and was immediately told to keep his head down. The assistant was still applying pressure to the incision and lifting the head affects the blood flowing through the artery. Rick said, "I want to go home tonight." I told the assistants and they sent us to the Cardiac Care Unit where we spent four hours with Rick flat on his back. I don't remember the drive home.

Tying Up Loose Ends
 I don't remember going to bed, but we got up the next

morning and Rick went in to work to turn over his case load and sign paperwork for a leave of absence. Rick came home and we remembered being asked for advance directives. We packed them along with a few things we thought Rick would need. I felt like we were watching a movie of ourselves in slow motion. It didn't seem real. We went over our agreement about DNR. Rick suggested several options regarding insurance monies and how I might best allocate them. We talked about the possibility of me moving to be close to my family if he did not survive the surgery. He did not want his family contacted before surgery and asked me not to contact them afterward. I could, however, contact his eldest sister. He told me to take care of myself first before distributing any monies. I felt like my ears were stuffed with cotton. I don't remember having any meals. I baked his favorite cookies.

I don't remember the drive to the hospital. I don't know how Rick was admitted. My next memory is of us sitting side by side on his bed like two little lost children. Rick's legs were crossed up on the bed and he was rocking back and forth. I was sitting with my legs dangling, staring off. I know we ate dinner, but I don't remember the meal. Two nurses came in and shaved Rick's body, they shaved his legs in case a vein needed to be harvested for repair work. I think Rick is a very hairy person, except for the top back of his head where you can see scalp. He was very pale without the dark curly hair. Already he was looking like a cadaver. I kept this thought to myself. "Don't voice it, it won't come true." The surgeon and the anesthesiologist visited us. A member from "Mended Hearts" came by. He gave us information for meetings and pulled me aside and said, "Be patient with him. He is going to say and do some very hurtful things during his recovery. Be patient." I was given the option to stay the night and sleep in a reclining chair. Rick and I thought it would be best for me to go home, get some sleep and a shower and return by 5 a.m. the next morning.

We were not counseled about the effects of open-chest heart surgery. We were not told about complications from bypass. We were told about anesthesia.

I don't remember leaving the hospital or going home. I remember walking into his room the next morning. He was cold and very nervous. The sedative was not working. He said he did not get much sleep even with medication. The operating room nurses arrived and we all rode together in the elevator to the operating room floor. Rick and I kissed and he said, "Bye-bye Rosie, find somebody nice." What a thing to say! What if that statement was the last I would remember of his voice! I was directed to the waiting room and told a nurse would keep me advised during surgery. I found a seat and tried to read. Somebody gave me a voucher for a free cup of coffee. I got coffee and tried to read again. Just where was that co-worker of Rick's who said she would clear her calendar and come sit with me? Notice of the surgery was so short that not one member of my family could get there in time. If they couldn't be there to see me through the surgery and possibility of Rick dying during the procedure, then I didn't want anyone there after the surgery. I wouldn't have time to spend with them, entertain them, feed them, or talk to them if he did survive. I knew he would consume all of my time. If he didn't survive, I didn't want anyone telling me what to do. Rick and I have been on our own since the beginning of our relationship and at the time of surgery, that was 17 years. We never asked for assistance in any way from either family, due to our family histories.

A nurse appeared and announced from the door, "Mrs. Froyd, is Mrs. Froyd here?" She told me Rick had been placed on bypass and the next time I would see her was when he would be off bypass. Now everyone in the waiting room knew too. I got those "I feel sorry for her" looks. So I sat and sat and waited and waited. The nurse appeared again and now knowing who Mrs. Froyd was, came up to me and told me Rick was off bypass and doing well, that his heart had started beating on its own. She told me to wait about one hour then to go to ICU to see him. I went up to ICU and waited in the chairs by the elevator. My friend from work stepped off the elevator and I was so glad to see someone I knew. I told people from work that there would be someone sitting with me during the surgery, so my friend waited until her lunch break to come see me. Rick's co-worker never showed. I was so disappointed. Rick felt sure someone would be with me and had told me that he had described me to her so that she would find me. My disappointment was for him and me. But then, Rick and I have only been able to depend on each other throughout our time together. This held true in this situation also.

It was 1:30 p.m. before I got to see Rick in ICU. The last time I had seen him was about 6 a.m. Fortunately, I knew what to expect as I had seen someone in ICU hooked up to all the monitors with tubes protruding from every possible site on the body. Still, it broke my spirit to see my big, fearless husband lying there so helpless. Rick tried very hard to come out of the anesthesia. His nurse was vigilant about his care and commented that she had never seen someone fight so hard to wake up. Each time Rick would open his eyes he tried to communicate, but he had tubes down his throat and nose and was tied down to the bed to avoid disconnecting the monitor cables. He was able to mouth, "I love you" to me several times and communicated in writing to the nurse about her concern when the alarm that went off. We kept telling him that the alarm would go off if he did not breathe on his own, so he needed to breath. He didn't seem to remember that we had told him that before. I watched him for about two hours, telling him his pulse and blood pressure and helping the nurse get him comfortable by letting her know that he needed to be straightened up. He tried to convey the message to her, but I understood right away. She was extremely proficient and caring. It might have seemed strange for someone to hear me reading off those numbers from the monitors, but Rick is the type of person that wants to know everything. I felt comfortable leaving for a short while to get something to eat.

When I returned a change of shift had taken place. The new nurse was nice and was caring for Rick very well. She informed me that some tubes would be removed later in the evening. About 10 p.m. she came up to me and told me I looked very tired and that I should go home and rest because Rick would need me more tomorrow. I left the hospital feeling that Rick was safe.

I returned the next morning to a new nurse. This nurse was not personable at all. I had to go out to the nurse's station several times to check on med times because Rick was not able to talk and was in pain. The nurse was not willing to help alleviate the pain in any way. He would not call the doctor. I had to go out and ask for a blanket because Rick was cold. When the nurse came in to check on Rick, he was not gentle or caring. He did not have the compassion of the previous nurses. It was most evident that he did not consider the patients to be humans with feelings and I had to pry information about Rick's condition out of him. He spoke to me as if I was bothering him and didn't understand anyway, so why should he waste his time. I did not feel good about leaving Rick with this nurse. I had to leave Rick in his charge because that male nurse was the one that would disconnect him and transfer Rick to the Cardiac Care Unit (CCU).

I went to the CCU floor, waited, and waited for Rick to come down. My friend from work stopped by again. It was good to see her and she brought messages from the office wishing me well and Rick a speedy recovery. Finally, Rick appeared and was settled into his room. He said the experience with the male nurse was not pleasant. Again, I urge that a person be with a patient as much as possible during the hospital stay. The patient has no one to depend on. Although the nursing and assistant staff on CCU were considerate and caring, the ratio was six patients to one nurse and two assistants. CCU patients cannot do anything for themselves for at least three days and even after that need assistance getting in and out of bed.

Recovery in the Hospital?
There is no such thing as recovering in the hospital. The hospital is to stabilize vital signs and medication dosages. There is very little time, if any, for patient's personal care. We learned this very quickly. Each day I visited with Rick, I was the one to sponge bathe him and wash and comb his hair. During the day, I cleaned his face with facial wipes and put lotion on his dry skin. I cut up his meals so he could feed himself and had to go in search of a nurse or assistant to help him get out of bed or to check on pain medication times. Unless it was time to check blood pressure, temperatures or administer meds, no one came to check on Rick.

"Mended Hearts" visited us again. They left information on their meetings. They did not ask how we were doing or if we needed any help. They did not counsel us on what to expect next in the recovery period. We heard, from nurses and patients that the third day after surgery was the worst. Still don't know why. My guess is that is when all the pain meds and anesthesia from the surgery have left the body. It proved to be true in our case.

Rick can be a most horrible person when he sets his mind to it. He did. He ordered everyone out of his room one day announcing that he was not going to eat, not going to walk, not going to cough, and told me to go home. Period. He scared the little nursing assistant and she went scurrying. She didn't tell the nurse that he was acting out. Rick again told me to leave, turned the thermostat up as high as it would go and went to sleep. I sat there for a while until the heat chased me out. I went down to the cafeteria had a nice dinner then went back up to CCU. On the way to his room, I stopped at the nurse's station. A change in shift had taken place and I found the new assistant. I told her what had happened. By this time, Rick had taken a nap for about two hours. I told the assistant that Rick was trying to die. Well that got her attention and she went charging into his room, told him to get ready to walk, turned down the thermostat and took him for a walk. I sat there, smiling, waiting for his return. His mood had improved immensely after his walk and talk with the assistant. He started acting better after that although complications set in.

Skilled Nursing Facility

Rick developed problems with his lungs due to asthma. He was transferred to the Skilled Nursing Facility. Rick told me his experiences on the floor were uncomfortable. I never spoke with staff in this department. It was as if there were no staff. This is Skilled Nursing? Rick took breathing treatments that were painful. He bathed himself and took care of his needs himself. He was supposed to meet with a nutritionist because of a change in diet. He needs to watch the amount of vitamin K in foods. The nutritionist was not able to give detailed information on that subject. You would think that they would come prepared with the patient's needs in mind and with useful information other than the food pyramid. I visited evenings because I had gone back to work. After nine days in the hospital, Rick was released.

The Long Road To Recovery

The first week home was an adjustment period for Rick getting used to his limitations. He had a Home Health nurse visit him every day for several weeks. He developed a good relationship with her and she was able to educate him about

INR levels and side effects of medications he was taking. She also told him how important it was for him to get up every day and shower and to dress in clothes, not to stay in pajamas.

Day by day and little by little, Rick was able to do more for himself. We expected him to get stronger as time passed but what we did not expect, and were not counseled to expect, were the possible mood changes that could occur. These mood changes were the most difficult of the recovery period for me. I cannot imagine the difficulty they caused Rick. This must have been what the person from Mended Hearts referred to when he advised me to be patient. I can say without doubt that only a few things kept me from leaving Rick during this trying period. These are my love for Rick that was built through the years, together facing obstacles and joys that life brings and caring for him as a human being with feelings, but most of all the strength that God gave me to believe that all would turn out well. The faith that that last item called for was the most difficult of all. I was not going to desert Rick in a time when he was vulnerable and needed to depend on someone. Rick developed an anger that was so strong that it was ugly and hurtful. He wanted to die. He wanted a divorce. He cut off almost every acquaintance. He refused to go out. He became a recluse, confined to the house and perimeter of our yard. Then he hit a high and went on a spending spree and days and nights of constant activity. I was afraid for him. I thought he was going to have a breakdown. I sought help from his former therapist. She put me off by that stupid "confidentiality" crap, even after I divulged I knew topics of their conversation and actually told her some in detail. All she did was inhale sharply and told me to contact his PCP. This PCP was professional and cared enough about me, as well as Rick, to talk to us both. The doctor prescribed a mood stabilizer and talked about a referral to a psychiatrist. I did not feel that the former therapist cared enough about Rick to also care about me and our situation.

After all, Rick and I were in this together, regardless that he had told her about wanting a divorce, he needed help and I was the only one here to give him that help. Against my advice, Rick allowed that therapist to talk him in to an inpatient psychiatric hospital on a voluntary basis. Even though I was against leaving him there, I went along with this venture in hopes that he would trust me. Trust me to believe in him and to try to get him help. He didn't last 24 hours. I went to pick him up, but his bad, angry moods persisted. I knew that the best place for Rick to recover was in his home, with his workout equipment, his music, his TV and movies, and me—the person who really cares about him. At that time, I didn't know if he was still serious about divorcing. I just knew that he needed someone on his side, every day, in every situation.

Helpful Contact Information

Rick Froyd
A web site dedicated to the personal experiences of the heart surgery survivor. A bi-weekly column is written on different aspects of living with heart disease from the patient's point of view

www.rickfroyd.org

The American Heart Association
They are a wonderful resource with plenty of great information.

National Center
7272 Greenville Avenue
Dallas, TX 75231-4596
www.americanheart.org
1 800 242 8721

The Heart Failure Society of America, Inc.
An excellent Web Site loaded with good information.

Executive Director: Cheryl Yeano
Court International, Suite 238N
2550 University Avenue West
St. Paul, MN 55114
www.hfsa.org
651 642 1633
651 642 1502 Fax
Cyano@hfsa.org

Studio-Delos

This web site has a listing of almost any support group that deals with medical issues that are out there. I have not personally looked at each link, but feel free to browse!

www.studio-delos

Mended Hearts

7272 Greenville Avenue
Dallas, Texas 75231
214 706 1442
214 706 5231
www.mendedhearts.org

References

American Heart Association. (1999). *Heart and Statistical Update*.

American Psychiatric Association. (1994). *Diagnostic and Statistical Manual of Mental Disorders* (4th ed.). Washington, D.C.

Kottler, J. A. (1991) *The Compleat Therapist*. San Francisco: Jossey-Bass, Inc., Publishers.

Lindsay, H. (1970) *The Late Great Planet Earth*.

Printed in the United States
18428LVS00001B/222